SCREENING FOR HEARING IMPAIRMENT IN YOUNG CHILDREN

Screening for Hearing Impairment in Young Children

Barry McCormick

Top Grade Audiological Scientist,
Director of the Children's Hearing Assessment Centre,
General Hospital, Nottingham

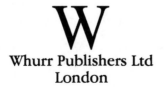

Whurr Publishers Ltd
London

First published 1988 by Chapman & Hall
Republished 1994 by Whurr Publishers Ltd
19b Compton Terrace, London N1 2UN, England

British Library Cataloguing in Publication Data
A catalogue record for this book is available from the
British Library.

ISBN 1-897635-66-4

Photoset by Mayhew Typesetting, Bristol
Printed and bound in the UK by Athenaeum Press Ltd,
Newcastle upon Tyne

Contents

Preface   vii

Introduction   ix

1. Basic Acoustics, the Hearing System and Causes
   of Deafness   1

2. The Concept of Hearing Screening and Basic Test
   Requirements   21

3. Utilising Parents' Suspicions: The Hints for
   Parents' Approach   39

4. The Modified Distraction Test for Babies between
   Six Months and Eighteen Months   44

5. Testing the Hearing of Children with Mental Ages
   between Eighteen Months and Two-and-a-Half
   Years   65

6. Testing the Hearing of Children with Mental Ages
   between Two-and-a-Half and Three-and-a-Half
   Years   75

7. The Sound-Level Meter and Room Acoustics   91

8. The Future — New Methods on the Horizon   98

References   105

Index   108

Preface

The serious effects of hearing impairment in children are generally not fully appreciated and hearing screening tests have rarely achieved an acceptable degree of reliability. For various reasons screening programmes have often failed to succeed in their function to provide onward referral for many cases of hearing impairment with the resulting consequence that the provision of help and treatment has been delayed.

It is often the exception rather than the norm for hearing problems to be detected within the first year of life. The average age for identification of congenital hearing impairment in children is in the region of 2–3 years and such late detection may restrict the degree to which the medical and educational services can maximise the potential of affected children.

The reasons why such poor standards have prevailed in traditional screening programmes are discussed in this book with reference to detailed analyses of service records from one county service in the United Kingdom. Suggestions for improving standards are then presented in the light of experience gained from applying new initiatives which have been shown to have a measured substantial effect on the record of success of the screening programme.

This book should be of general interest to anyone engaged in professional work with children and it contains advice of direct practical significance for those who are responsible for screening the hearing of children. It must, however, be stated at the onset that no text can impart practical skills to the reader for such skills can only be developed with the benefit of expert supervision in a practical training context. Furthermore it is apparent that many people are forming opinions about babies' and children's development and linguistic skills without knowledge of whether progress is being influenced by a hearing disorder. In view of this reality it is hoped that this book will make a significant contribution by highlighting first, the need for hearing screening and secondly, the essential minimum requirements for hearing screening programmes.

No attempt is made in this book to review in detail hearing test methods which require large capital expenditure on equipment. The semi or fully automated tests now available, mostly for neonatal screening programmes, are being researched and evaluated by the writer and his colleagues and by other teams in the world and they will no doubt find widespread use in years to come. Currently they are confined to use within research programmes and it is the method and instrumentation which is subject to evaluation as much as the child. Whatever developments occur in the hi-tech field there will always be the need to apply the type of behavioural screen presented in detail in this book. Whether the new technology will be used to back up the behavioural methods or vice versa will be a subject for debate for some time to come.

Introduction

Unlike many disabling conditions hearing impairment does not have any overtly visible feature to the lay person, or even to doctors or other professional people. The problems faced by blind or physically disabled individuals can be appreciated at least to some degree, and this immediate awareness tends to attract constructive support from the general public. This is not so for the hearing impaired for they are often mistakenly considered to be retarded. The invisible nature of this disabling condition is such that it strikes at the heart of the communication system used by humans affecting not only receptive and expressive language facility but also possible social and emotional development.

One feature of hearing impairment not widely appreciated is that the severity of the sensory loss can be of any degree from very slight to very profound. At one extreme a child with a temporary fluctuating conductive hearing loss of minor degree might appear to be only slightly inconvenienced, although some studies have demonstrated resulting retardation in linguistic and educational progress in addition to associated behaviour problems; examples are presented by Dalzell and Owrid (1976), Downs (1981), Hamilton (1972), Paradise (1983) and Jerger, Jerger, Alford and Abrams (1983). At the other extreme the severely or profoundly congenitally deafened child may fail to acquire speech and language skills unless special help, in the form of hearing-aid provision and language stimulation programmes, is provided at a very early stage.

Another feature of hearing impairment which may not be appreciated is that certain frequencies may be heard quite well and others not at all or only in a very distorted fashion. For example, a child with a high tone hearing loss may not hear the clarity of higher frequency speech sounds such as the sibilants but may hear lower frequency sounds in speech. A child with this condition may, for example, be able to hear a pin drop but speech may sound very indistinct due to the omission or distortion of certain sounds. It is not unknown for children with an undiagnosed form of this condition to be misdiagnosed as slow learners or even educationally subnormal despite normal or above normal intellectual ability.

It is vital, because of the hidden nature of the problem, that an active detection strategy should be employed. If this approach is not adopted, hearing problems may be detected only when the more obvious signs become manifest in the child's behaviour and development and, by then, irreversible damage may have been done. It is particularly important to detect congenital hearing problems during the early months of life because it is known that certain important language features should be experienced by the baby in the critical first year of life. Failure to gain from these experiences can have serious consequences (Tervoort, 1964; Menyuk, 1977; Boothman and Orr, 1978; Gerber and Mencher, 1978; Rapin, 1978). There is, in fact, a strong probability that lack of sensory stimulation in the early critical stages can produce irreversible neurological changes which may limit subsequent development. This has certainly been shown to be the case with animals and the circumstantial evidence of the extreme difficulties faced by children whose hearing impairments are detected late supports the notion that the same may apply to human subjects. It is certainly evident that congenitally deafened children experience much greater difficulty in acquiring speech and language skills than their peers who become deaf within the second or third year of life.

Although the need for early detection is well defined, the current state of routine hearing screening practice is far from ideal. Martin and Moore (1979) and Martin, Bentzen, Golley, Hennebert, Holm, Iurato, de Jonge, McCullen, Meyer, Moore and Morgan (1981) reported data collected from the EEC countries which confirmed that only 10 per cent of hearing-impaired children had their condition detected in the first year of life and 50 per cent of the children with an average hearing loss of 50dB or more in the better ear had passed their third birthday before the deafness was confirmed. According to Simmons (1978) the national age-average for detection of hearing loss in the United States of America is 2.7 years. Detailed analysis of the records from the county of Nottinghamshire in England (prior to the introduction of new initiatives to improve the system) confirmed this same trend of late detection (McCormick, Wood, Cope and Spavins, 1984). It is apparent that the general situation has not shown any major improvement in recent years except in a few areas where more intensive training of screeners and more rigorous screening techniques have been introduced.

The techniques which have been tried, evaluated, and routinely applied in Nottinghamshire with good effect will be described fully in this book.

1

Basic Acoustics, the Hearing System and Causes of Deafness

Sound is defined as any pressure variation (in air, water or some other medium) that the human ear can detect. The human hearing system has evolved to respond to a wide range of sounds in the environment but it functions at its peak of sensitivity to those sounds in the human speech range.

Sound can be characterised by three main features, namely, intensity, frequency, and duration. Intensity is perceived as loudness and frequency as pitch and these, together with the ability to comprehend speech, are the main characteristic features which we attempt to check in simple forms of hearing tests. There are other complex interactions which can be measured in more sophisticated diagnostic hearing tests, for example temporal processing (time relationships) and frequency resolution (or separation). Consideration of these is, however, beyond the scope of this book because simple 'screening' methods have not yet been devised for measuring these characteristics in a form suitable for routine application with babies and children.

Returning to basics, sound is produced by vibrations and these vibrations may be characterised by their rapidity and force (or pressure) which, in turn, will determine the pitch and loudness of the sensation produced in the hearing system. The picture can begin to unfold by taking each of these in turn.

PITCH

The young healthy normal ear can perceive as pitch a wide range of frequencies from approximately 20 pressure variations per second (20 Hertz or Hz) at the lower end up to 20,000 pressure variations

1

Table 1.1: Frequency spectra (approximate)

Man	20 Hz– 20 kHz
Dog	15 Hz– 50 kHz
Cat	60 Hz– 65 kHz
Dolphin	150 Hz–150 kHz
Bat	1 kHz–120 kHz
Piano	30 Hz– 4 kHz

per second (20 kHz) at the upper limit (Table 1.1). Pressure variations outside these ranges do exist, of course, but they do not stimulate the hearing pathway of man. Viewed in physical terms they have a frequency but are not perceived as having a pitch for man. Bats, for example, can perceive vibrations up to 120 kHz and dolphins extend the range even further up to 150 kHz. A relatively limited range of frequencies available to man is actually used in speech and most of the sounds in speech occur in the frequency range from 250 Hz up to 8 kHz. This range can be reduced even to 500 Hz–4 kHz without producing any serious deterioration in the clarity of speech. The piano offers a useful reference for the frequency scale with the lowest note having a frequency of 27.5 Hz and the highest note having a frequency of 4,186 Hz. Middle C has a frequency of 256 Hz.

For convenience, only certain frequencies are used for hearing measurement purposes and these are chosen such that each is taken as either double or half the adjacent value. The lowest frequency of interest for speech and hearing purposes is usually 125 Hz and subsequent ones are taken at octave intervals above this, the octave being a doubling of frequency. The frequency scale appears as follows:

125 Hz, 250 Hz, 500 Hz, 1 kHz, 2 kHz, 4 kHz, 8 kHz

Higher frequencies above 8 kHz may occasionally be considered and also mid-octave intervals such as 750 Hz, 1.5 kHz, 3 kHz and 6 kHz may sometimes be of interest.

LOUDNESS

The human ear is responsive to a wide range of sound pressures and the difference between the pressure of the quietest sound which can

Figure 1.1: The decibel scale

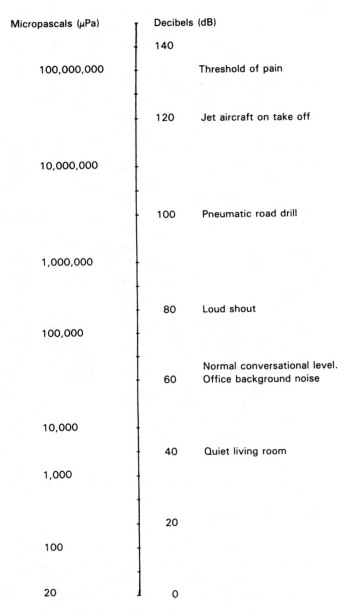

be heard and the loudest sound which can be tolerated is several million-fold. To accommodate this vast range of values on a convenient scale with simple notation a logarithmic scale is used with a basic unit known as the decibel (dB). An illustration of typical decibel values of everyday sounds is given in Figure 1.1. It can be seen that the decibel scale compresses the million to one pressure values into a 0–120dB range.

For convenience (although adding to confusion) different decibel scales are used according to the area of interest. Such scales include the dB(A), dB(B), dB(C), dB(D), dB(Hearing Level or HL) and dB(Sound Pressure Level or SPL) scales. The reason why such a range of scales exists is that the human ear is not equally sensitive to all frequencies and this sensitivity changes as the sound pressure increases. For quiet sound the human ear is most sensitive in the frequency range between 2 kHz and 5 kHz and is least sensitive at extremely high and low frequencies. For louder sounds the differences in sensitivity are not so great. The different decibel scales attempt to characterise the way this sensitivity changes. The scales used almost exclusively for hearing screening purposes are the dB(A) and dB(HL). dB(A) is used when a sound level is being measured in a room setting and dB(HL) is used when sounds are presented through earphones. The two scales differ by 4dB or so depending upon the frequency of the sound in question with the dB(A) values being higher numerically. The reference value of 0dB ISO (International Organisation for Standardisation) corresponds to the quietest level at which young healthy normally hearing subjects can just hear a sound on two out of three of the occasions when it is presented. This is an average value and it is possible for some individuals to hear at even quieter levels of −10 dB or even −20 dB.

AN INTRODUCTION TO THE PURE TONE AUDIOGRAM

The pure tone audiogram is a convenient chart for recording the threshold levels at which an individual listening through standard earphones can hear different frequencies known as pure tones (because they contain a single or pure frequency of pressure variation). The basic audiogram scale configuration is shown in Figure 1.2. The frequency scale covers the range from 125 Hz up to 8 kHz along the horizontal (abscissa) axis and the vertical (ordinate) hearing-level scale covers the range from −20 dB(HL) (ISO) up to 120 dB(HL) (ISO). To establish the audiometric threshold at each

Figure 1.2: The audiogram

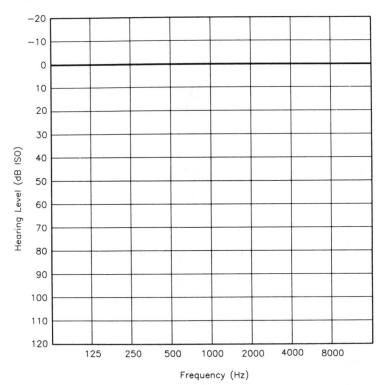

frequency it is necessary to follow a standard procedure and it is not appropriate to discuss this fully in the context of an introduction to a screening system.

Examples of audiometric configurations are shown in Figure 1.3. Figure 1.3(i) shows the audiogram for the right (o) and left (x) ears of a person with normal hearing and Figure 1.3(ii) shows the pattern for a person with a flat 30 dB hearing loss. Figure 1.3(iii) shows the audiogram for somebody with a flat 60 dB hearing loss in the left ear and a more severe or profound hearing loss in excess of 100 dB in the right ear. Figure 1.3(iv) shows the audiogram of a person with a high tone hearing loss who can hear low and middle speech frequencies at normal levels but the hearing for the high frequencies is significantly impaired. In a case such as this the affected person will not hear some of the higher frequency sounds in speech and other speech sounds will appear distorted because they lack the high

Figure 1.3: Examples of audiogram configurations (air conduction only)

(i) Normal hearing

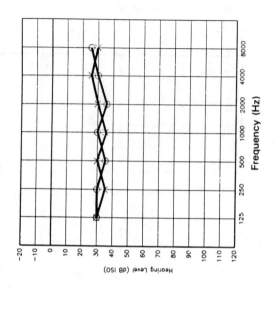

(ii) Flat 30dBHL bilateral hearing loss

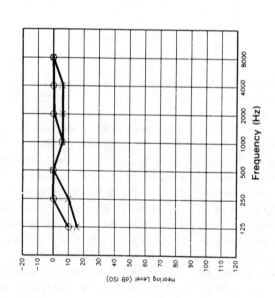

Figure 1.3 *continued*

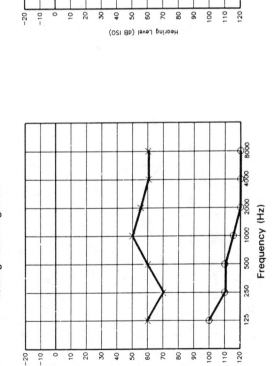

(iii) Flat 60dBHL hearing loss in left ear, severe/profound hearing loss in right ear

(iv) High tone hearing loss

Figure 1.3 *continued*

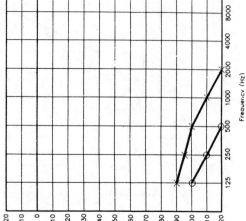

(v) Moderate unilateral hearing loss

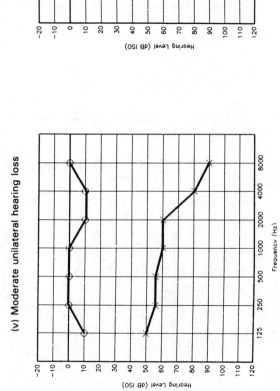

(vi) Profound bilateral hearing loss

frequency components.

Figure 1.3(v) shows the audiogram of somebody with a moderate unilateral hearing loss of 60/70 dB in the left ear and Figure 1.3(vi) shows a typical example of a profound bilateral hearing loss. The above discussion relates only to what is known as *air conduction audiometry*, that is the recording of hearing thresholds using earphones positioned on the ears. It is possible to record hearing thresholds by means of a vibrator placed on the skull, usually on the mastoid bone behind the ear. In this case pure tone *threshold for bone conducted sounds* can be recorded. The following introduction to the basic anatomy of the ear and of the way in which it functions will help to clarify the situation.

AN INTRODUCTION TO THE HEARING SYSTEM

A simplified diagram of the hearing system is shown in Figure 1.4. Sound waves (in the form of pressure variations) enter the outer ear canal (external auditory meatus) where they meet the eardrum (tympanic membrane). The eardrum is, in effect, a tightly stretched area of skin rather like the membrane of a drum. The eardrum is set into vibration when the sound strikes it. Attached to the eardrum is the first of three bones (the ossicles) which are linked together and span the air-filled space called the middle ear cavity. The vibrations from the eardrum are transmitted across the middle ear by these bones which act as a set of levers. The effect is to create a powerful vibration of the last bone in the linked chain, the stapes, which is embedded in another membrane, the oval window. Beyond the oval window is a complex fluid-filled system (the cochlea) containing the nerves of hearing. The vibration of the stapes in the oval window creates a rocking plunger action which sets the fluid in the cochlea into vibration. It is the movement of this vibrating fluid which activates the nerves within the cochlea, giving rise to impulses which are passed along the auditory nerve pathways to the auditory areas of the brain where the signals are interpreted and given meaning.

From this simplified description of the main essentials of the system it is apparent that the hearing mechanism involves mechanical movements or vibration in addition to nerve function. Anything which impedes the passage of vibrations along the outer or middle ear structures will produce a *conductive hearing loss*. Otitis media is the most common disorder of this nature and in this case the presence of mucus fluid in the middle ear space, secreted

9

Figure 1.4: Schematic diagram of the ear (not to scale)

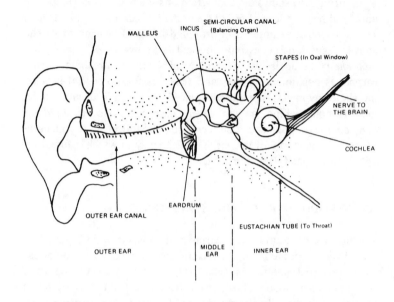

from the mucus membrane lining, restricts the movements of the ossicular chain and the eardrum. The resulting hearing loss may be of any severity up to a maximum of 60 dB. The maximum severity for any type of conductive hearing loss is, in fact, 60 dB because sounds may still penetrate through to the oval window either by bone and tissue vibration (in the case of blockage) or by air-borne vibrations in the case of the absence of the tympanic membrane and ossicular chain structure. When a vibrator is placed on the mastoid bone the vibrations pass directly to the oval window through the bone structure thereby bypassing the outer and middle ear structures. The hearing thresholds recorded from a bone vibrator (that is the bone conduction thresholds) will be normal in the case of a conductive hearing loss but the air-conducted thresholds will be elevated. An example of the audiometric configuration for a typical conductive hearing loss is given in Figure 1.5. Notice the use of a triangular symbol for bone conduction thresholds recorded without masking (that is without excluding one of the ears from the test by occupying it with a noise). The signal produced from a vibrator placed anywhere on the skull will be transmitted through the structures to both cochleae with little transcranial attenuation. It is, therefore, impossible to know whether one or both cochleae are

10

Figure 1.5: Typical audiometric configuration for a conductive hearing impairment

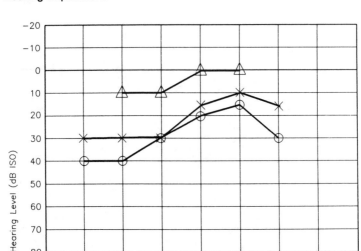

responding unless a procedure of masking is undertaken in which one ear is occupied with a carefully selected narrow band noise to exclude it from the threshold determination. This masking procedure is too involved for discussion in this text on screening but the interested reader can find a simple discussion of the general principles in Tucker and Nolan (1984). The difference between the air-conduction and bone-conduction thresholds is known as the air-bone gap and this gives an indication of the extent of the conductive hearing impairment.

If bone-conduction thresholds are depressed then clearly there is some dysfunction beyond the middle ear, and hearing problems which result from damage to the cochlear structures and nerve parts of the hearing system are called *sensori-neural hearing impairments*. They can be caused by any disease state which interrupts the supply

11

Figure 1.6: Typical audiometric configuration for a sensori-neural hearing impairment

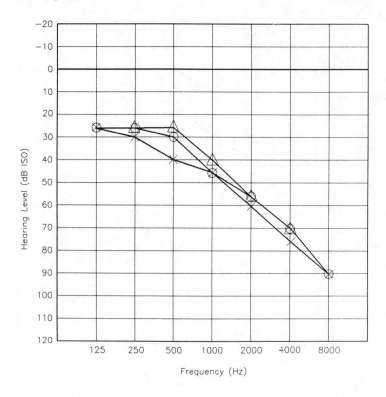

of essential nutrients to the nerves, or which interferes with the conduction of nerve impulses. An audiometric configuration for a sensori-neural hearing impairment is given in Figure 1.6.

MAIN CAUSES OF HEARING LOSS

It is not the intention in this book to review the causes of deafness in detail. Excellent accounts have been given by Fraser (1976), Jaffe (1977) and Northern and Downs (1982). Some of the most commonly related factors are presented below.

Conductive hearing loss

Any swelling or foreign body which completely blocks the external auditory meatus can cause a conductive hearing loss but such occurrence is fairly rare, with the exception of the build up of wax or the insertion of objects in the ear by children. In nearly all cases the obstruction can be cleared, thereby restoring normal hearing. If the tympanic membrane becomes damaged or perforated this may cause some degree of hearing problem until it is repaired by, for example, myringoplasty operation (surgical reconstruction of the drum).

Conductive hearing loss in the middle ear may result from disruption or fixation of the ossicular chain system or from the presence of fluid in the middle ear which restricts the vibration motion of the system (for example secretory otitis media). In most cases conductive hearing losses of the above type can be cleared either with medical or surgical treatment or, in some cases, by spontaneous remission.

In the bone disease known as otosclerosis, the stapes becomes fixed in the oval window with subsequent impairment of its normal vibration. Conductive losses due to this can sometimes be alleviated by surgical replacement of the diseased bone by a prosthetic structure. Otosclerosis is, however, rare in the very young child.

There are, of course, other forms of conductive hearing loss due to abnormalities of the middle ear structures caused by accidents or by failure of the system to develop properly, and in some of these cases the damage or malformation may not be correctable by surgery. Middle ear anomalies might be present whenever other branchial arch anomalies are observed. The most observable or apparent feature might be atresia of the external auditory canal and low set or absent auricles. Middle ear malformations may exist in cases of osteogenesis imperfecta, Treacher-Collin's syndrome, Pierre Robin syndrome, cleft palate, Apert's syndrome, Klippel Feil syndrome, Crouzon's syndrome (cranio-facial dysostosis), Paget's disease, van der Hoeve's disease, and Goldenhar's syndrome.

Otitis media

Acute suppurative otitis media. This condition is extremely common in the pre-school years with 80 per cent of children having at least one attack prior to the age of 5 years; it is often associated with nasopharyngitis. The Eustachian tube of infants is shorter and more horizontal than that of adults, thus increasing the chance of infection spreading to the middle ear space. Conductive hearing loss

13

associated with this condition results from the presence of pus from the swollen infected lining of the middle ear space. In severe cases the drum bursts and the pus is released: in the majority of cases of acute otitis media the inflammatory conditions clears after a few days, often aided by antibiotic treatment. The conductive hearing loss should then resolve as ventilation is restored to the middle ear space. It is possible, however, for the fluid to remain and the hearing loss may persist.

Serous otitis media (glue ear). Conductive hearing loss originates in this condition due to the presence of fluid in the middle ear but this condition differs from acute otitis media by virtue of the fact that the fluid is sterile. In a few cases there may be a positive allergy history and in some cases the condition appears to be an aftermath of an attack of acute otitis media, particularly after antibiotic treatment. The condition develops due to inadequate ventilation of the middle ear through the Eustachian tube. Reabsorption of air within the middle ear produces the negative pressure within the space and consequent retraction of the tympanic membrane plus secretion of a transudate from the mucous membrane lining. This fluid later becomes mucoid or exudative in consistency especially when the disorder is of long duration.

Serous otitis media may persist for many months or even years if untreated and the associated hearing loss, often in the region of 30–50 dB, may vary widely. The low frequency thresholds (below 1 kHz) are affected initially and then the high frequencies (above 2 kHz) and finally the mid-frequencies centred on 2 kHz. Sometimes even if fluid is present the hearing may be normal.

Although serous otitis media will eventually resolve itself it may be necessary to intervene to avoid educational and behavioural problems. Treatment may consist, in the first instance, of courses of decongestants and/or antihistamines or Septrin (an antibacterial drug). For persistent cases the surgeon may ventilate the middle ear by making an incision in the tympanic membrane and removing the pus by suction (myringotomy operation). In some instances a grommet may be inserted in the incision to maintain a ventilation effect for several months until the Eustachian tube returns to normal function. Adenoidectomy may also be indicated to prevent the development of further effusions.

It is important that parents (and teachers) should be aware of the presence and fluctuating nature of the hearing impairment. The writer's advice sheet shown in Figure 1.7 has proved to be

Figure 1.7: Nottinghamshire Children's Hearing Assessment Centre Advisory Document No. 2

ADVICE FOR PARENTS AND TEACHERS CONCERNING CHILDREN WITH HEARING PROBLEMS OF A MINOR DEGREE

A child with a slight hearing problem may not need or even be able to benefit from a hearing aid but, nevertheless, he or she may be at risk both in terms of language development and in terms of educational progess. It is hoped that the advice given below will help parents and teachers to form some appreciation of the nature of the child's problems and this may help to lessen the risk to the child.

The Child's Problems

1. It is important to understand that the child's main problem is not lack of awareness of sound for in certain circumstances even very quiet sounds may be heard. The problem is more one of sound confusion because some parts of speech may be heard less well than others. The child may be aware of a very quiet voice or even a whisper but he or she may miss the clarity of the speech. Some words may be missed altogether and others may be confused.

2. It is highly likely that a child with this degree of hearing disorder will have been accused of being rather slow or inattentive when in fact the child has a genuine problem in making sense of what is said.

3. The child's problem will be much greater in noisy surroundings or in situations where more than one person is speaking at the same time.

4. The hearing levels may fluctuate from day to day. On good days the child's hearing may appear to be virtually normal and on poor days the child may have considerable difficulty.

5. If one ear is affected more than the other the child may experience difficulty in locating sounds and in understanding speech presented on the poor side.

What Parents and Teachers Should Do

1. Careful thought should be given to seating arrangements in classrooms or to the distance at which speech is presented to the child in other situations. The speaker should attempt to be as near as possible to the child and be on the better side if one ear is affected more than the other.

2. The child will be helped if he or she can see the speaker's face.

3. Patience may be needed if the child repeatedly misunderstands.

Dr. B. McCormick PhD, BSc, Cert. T. Deaf, Dip. Audiol.
Director of the Children's Hearing Assessment Centre.

extremely useful for this purpose.

Cholesteatoma

Another condition which may cause a conductive hearing impairment is cholesteatoma. This denotes an abnormal presence of skin in the middle ear or mastoid, usually occurring due to the accumulation of epithelial growth within a retraction pocket of the tympanic membrane. Expansion of the cholesteatoma may restrict the movement of the tympanic membrane and eventually destroy the membrane, the ossicles, the bony walls of the cochlea, and other structures. If unchecked this uncommon condition can be life threatening due to the development of intracranial complications such as a brain abscess.

Sensori-neural hearing loss

It is convenient to classify sensori-neural hearing impairments into two categories, namely, congenital and acquired. By far the greatest proportion of cases have a congenital origin and the following have been cited as factors.

1. Congenital

   Genetic conditions (family history of deafness)
   Maternal rubella
   Cytomegalovirus
   Meningitis
   Rhesus incompatibility
   Inherited otosclerosis
   Ototoxic drugs taken by the mother during pregnancy
   Prematurity
   Brain damage (e.g. cerebral palsy).

2. Acquired

   Meningitis/Encephalitis
   Other infectious diseases (measles, mumps, smallpox, scarlet fever)
   Ototoxic drugs
   Head trauma
   Acoustic nerve tumour (neuromas)

16

Ménière's disease

Stroke.

Genetic

It is estimated that there may be about 150 genetic disorders linked with deafness and it is not surprising that genetic factors are indicated in at least one half of all cases of deafness. Many of the cases in which no known cause of deafness can be found may have a genetic origin.

There are three classifications for genetic inheritance, namely, autosomal dominant, autosomal recessive and sex-linked. In the dominant conditions only one parent need carry the gene responsible for deafness and the chances of offspring being affected are 1 in 2. In the recessive condition both parents must be carriers and the chance of producing affected offspring is 1 in 4. Expert genetic counselling will be needed to give precise chance figures. In the case of sex-linked conditions the problem originates due to some abnormality in the X and Y chromosomes.

Deafness is sometimes one of a group of characteristics which form a syndrome. An example of a dominant condition of this nature is *Waardenburg syndrome* which accounts for 2 per cent of all congenitally deaf children. The features noted in the syndrome, in addition to sensori-neural deafness, include a white forelock, irises of two colours (heterochromia iridis), hyperplasia of medial portion of eyebrows, lateral displacement of medial canthi. The hearing impairment may be unilateral or bilateral and it may be progressive. In *Treacher-Collin's syndrome* (mandibulofacial dysostosis or first arch syndrome) deafness is mostly conductive in nature, although there may be a sensori-neural element in some cases. In this condition the external ears may be small and displaced and there may be atresia of the external auditory canal. In addition, the middle ear is often poorly developed with deformation or absence of the ossicles and other structures. Other visible features include facial bone abnormalities with downward sloping palpebral fissures, depressed cheek bones, receding chin, and large fish-like mouth with dental abnormalities.

Other examples of autosomal dominant conditions associated with sensorineural deafness include *Apert's syndrome* (acrocephalosyndactyly), *Alport's syndrome, Klippel-Feil syndrome, osteogenesis imperfecta* (brittle bone disease), *branchio oto-renal syndrome*, and *Crouzon's syndrome*.

Alport's disease is characterised by progressive nephritis with haematuria and proteinuria beginning in early childhood and often resulting in renal failure in early adult life. A progressive sensorineural hearing loss usually becomes established by ten years of age. *Pendred's syndrome* is an example of a recessive condition and in this case congenital deafness is associated with goitre appearing during adolescence.

In *Klippel-Feil syndrome* the affected child may show congenital sensori-neural deafness alongside fusion or reduction in the number of cervical vertebrae, a short neck, low hair line and limited neck movement.

Usher's syndrome is an example of a recessive condition associated with deafness and progressive visual disorder (retinitis pigmentosa). The visual disorders are of later onset than the deafness and often the first symptoms are night blindness and tunnel vision. Deafness in this, like most recessive conditions, is usually very severe or profound. It is estimated that between 5 and 10 per cent of all congenitally deafened children could have this condition and it is vital, therefore, that effective vision testing programmes should be available, in addition to hearing testing throughout the early years of childhood.

Cockayne syndrome is another autosomal recessive condition associated with progressive deterioration of hearing and progressive mental retardation. Hearing is usually normal at birth prior to the development of a progressive sensori-neural hearing loss. Other characteristic features include dwarfism with sensile 'pinched in' facial appearance.

Perhaps the most familiar X-linked syndrome associated with deafness is *Hunter's syndrome*. This disorder is not always apparent at birth but during the early months progressive abnormal traits appear including short stature, coarse facial features, and depressed nasal bridge. Later features include enlarged head, prominent eyebrows, thick lips, prominent abdomen, mental decline, blindness, and deafness. The deafness is conductive and/or sensori-neural and of moderate degree in the early stages but this may be progressive. Only males are affected by Hunter's syndrome.

No discussion of syndromes would be complete without the inclusion of *Down's syndrome*. Well over half of all cases of Down's syndrome will have serous otitis media associated with a long history of upper respiratory tract infections and middle ear infections. A small proportion will have mixed losses. Owing to the persistence of the conductive condition, often despite surgical and medical treatment, the option of hearing-aid fitting in the early years should be given serious consideration. Another group of children susceptible to serous otitis media is those with *cleft palate*. As with the Down's syndrome group the conductive hearing loss with cleft palate children is particularly prevalent (50–65 per cent) and intractable to treatment. Regular audiological assessment will be needed to assess the need for hearing aid provision.

Congenital causes other than genetic

Maternal rubella contracted during the first 3 months of pregnancy can produce devastating effects on the developing embryo, including deafness, blindness, mental disorders and heart lesions. The sensorineural deafness is usually severe in nature. Thanks to the programme of immunisation of school girls the disease has been contained and the number of babies affected has dropped dramatically in the past decade. Isolated cases do, however, still appear and there is some evidence that the condition is affecting a number of Asian babies. There is certainly a need for greater uptake of the immunisation programme.

Cytomegalovirus is another intrauterine infection, which is increasingly recognised and can cause severe or profound sensorineural hearing impairment and may be progressive in nature.

Caution will always be necessary when prescribing drugs for mothers during pregnancy for fear of ototoxicity. Potentially ototoxic drugs given to babies in the newborn period have included streptomycin, gentamycin, kanamycin, and colistin, and if given at all the doses must be very carefully monitored.

A high incidence of hearing loss has been reported in *premature babies* with the incidence being approximately ten times greater than for normal-term babies. *Respiratory distress, recurrent apnoeic* attacks, and *anoxia* have been cited as factors but the explanation of the situation is not clear-cut. It is known, however, that *hyperbilirubinaemia* can have a particularly toxic effect on the dorsal cochlea nuclei in the brainstem producing a high-tone hearing impairment.

The once common condition of *rhesus haemolitic disease* (incompatibility), which at one time accounted for some 10 per cent of all cases of deafness, has been brought under control thanks to the use of anti-D gamma-globulin. Prompt exchange transfusions and phototherapy treatment have reduced the number of cases of deafness due to neonatal hyperbilirubinaemia.

Acquired

Acquired or postnatal causes of sensori-neural hearing impairment include *meningitis* which may damage the auditory (8th) nerve, and *encephalitis* which may involve the cochlear nuclei and tracts in the brainstem. Mumps is a common cause of unilateral sensori-neural hearing loss, presumably due to labyrinthitis occurring at the time of the illness.

Severe *head injuries* in childhood may be associated with basal fractures involving the temporal bones and, therefore, lead to deafness.

Despite extensive investigation the cause of deafness often remains obscure although recessive deafness may be implicated. Most studies quote the proportion of unknown causes to be between 30 and 60 per cent.

SUMMARY

The complexities of sound and speech perception are such that not all aspects can be assessed in screening programmes. Two features of sound frequency and intensity, and their hearing correlates pitch and loudness, have been described.

The main causes of conductive and sensori-neural hearing loss have been presented and although the list of known causes is quite extensive the proportion of cases of unknown cause is still very high at between 30 and 60 per cent.

2

The Concept of Hearing Screening and Basic Test Requirements

Screening may be likened to fishing a flowing stream with a net the size of which must be adjusted to suit the intended catch. If the mesh of the net is too fine a large quantity of unnecessary catch will be made which will cause considerable time wastage at the sorting stage. Conversely, a large mesh will fail to catch all but the largest of the desired fish. Similarly the hearing screen must, by design, catch affected cases and let the unaffected cases pass through the system unhindered. Clearly a compromise approach is called for because a test which is too stringent would waste expensive follow-up resource by overloading it with unnecessary cases. The screening programme will also waste resource if it does not filter out the affected cases effectively. A good hearing screening programme will, through its administration, filter out from the population a fairly small target group of cases likely to exhibit a hearing disorder and it should do this with a high degree of sensitivity (that is, it should efficiently catch the affected cases) together with a high degree of specificity (that is, it should correctly release or identify unaffected cases). The formulae for quantifying these two descriptors of validity are:

$$\text{sensitivity} = \frac{a}{a+c}$$

$$\text{specificity} = \frac{d}{b+d}$$

where a = impairment present, test positive; b = impairment absent, test positive; c = impairment present, test negative; d = impairment absent, test negative.

Reference to Table 2.1 may make the situation clearer. The ideal

Table 2.1: Definition of sensitivity and specificity for screening studies

Screen result	Verified disease state	
	Disease	No disease
FAIL (positive)	True positive (a)	False positive (b)
PASS (negative)	False negative (c)	True negative (d)
	Sensitivity = (a)/(a) + (c)	Specificity = (d)/(d) + (b)

sensitivity is to find 100 per cent of those affected by hearing impairment and the ideal specificity would correctly classify 100 per cent of those not having an impairment. The ideal is, however, never achieved and a more realistic objective might be to aim for a sensitivity of 90 per cent and a specificity of 90 per cent, that is 1 in 10 with an impairment would be missed and 1 in 10 of those caught by the net would have normal hearing. The adverse consequences to those with impairment missed by the screen will be greater than the consequences to those incorrectly caught, for in the former case the screen may lead to delayed diagnosis whereas in the latter case the screen will simply waste follow-up resources. The two measures quoted for describing this aspect of the performance of the screen are the *false negative* and *false positive* values, where the false negative refers to the proportion of impaired cases not identified and the false positive (or false alarm) value refers to the proportion of normal cases caught incorrectly in the screening net.

The formulae for calculating these values using the above notation are:

$$\text{false negative proportion} = \frac{c}{a+c}$$

$$\text{false positive proportion} = \frac{b}{b+d}$$

The above are measures of validity for the screening test. A further measure is that of the reliability of the test and this is usually assessed by calculating correlation coefficients for repeated test results.

Unfortunately, in the field of hearing screening, very few studies have presented full and accurate data to support the validity and reliability of the test methods used. In an attempt to redress this situation the author and his colleagues have undertaken a detailed analysis of the distraction test and a series of papers is being prepared for publication. Sensitivity and specificity values of 80 per cent have been achieved with the distraction test following the incorporation of new initiatives and better training. These values are very much higher than the previous ones of between 10 per cent and 20 per cent referred to earlier in this book.

Clearly such measures are important for planning effective allocation of resource according to the efficiency of the method used. It is important that a clear distinction and separation should be made between a *screening* test and a test of *confirmation* (often termed the diagnostic test). The screening test is only the first stage in the process of identification which ultimately leads to confirmation. The screening test does not and should not confirm the presence or degree of any disorder but rather it should be a relatively simple and economical means whereby cases likely to have a certain degree of disorder are filtered out from the population and steered along a pathway to confirmation. Note here that the 'certain degree of disorder' is something that has to be specified in advance and the choice of this at the onset may be somewhat arbitrary. It may be, for example, that the objective is to filter out children with an average hearing loss in excess of 25 dB, in which case the assumption that those children exhibiting losses of less than or equal to 25 dB are not significantly impaired has to be accepted (rightly or wrongly). This arbitrary decision must be made on the basis of the screening programme's objectives.

When correctly applied a screening test should be performed at a set time, usually at a certain age, and it should cover a defined subpopulation of that age with an identical procedure. The term screening is, however, often used in a much more general sense to imply a simple test or a battery of tests applied in a surveillance context. Private health screening schemes and breast screening programmes are examples of health care systems which utilise the term screening in this context. In Great Britain it is normal to test the hearing of all babies in their first year of life and in most authorities it is a requirement that such tests be undertaken. The term screening can be used correctly in this context. Not all authorities have a routine system for testing the hearing of children between the ages of one year and five years, and those who do have a test available often use it in a surveillance rather than a screening context, that is, the test is only applied if certain pointers indicate its need. If the indicators are well defined and are based on quantifiable measures then they could be used to define the sub-population precisely. Unfortunately, the indicators are often somewhat vague and inaccessible to detailed quantification: 'delayed speech and language' and 'parental concern' are the most useful factors quoted. If the definition of the sub-group is somewhat vague and unquantifiable the term surveillance may be more appropriate than screening; sieving is even more apt.

THE OBJECTIVES OF HEARING SCREENING PROGRAMMES

Clearly the criteria set for the screen will depend upon the focus of interest.

If the hearing screening programme is to achieve its objective it should, through its application, refer onward not only the more serious cases with sensori-neural hearing loss but also the more common but less severe cases with conductive hearing loss. Preliminary analysis of data from the Nottingham district has indicated that for every baby with confirmed sensori-neural hearing loss in the first year of life there will be approximately 40 with persistent conductive hearing loss. The distraction test, when properly applied, can detect both groups. It is known that attacks of acute otitis media are highly prevalent in babies between the ages of 6 and 24 months (Klein, Bess, Bluestone and Harford, 1978) and approximately 75 per cent of acute otitis occurs before the age of one year (Pukander, Karma and Sipila, 1982). Isolated attacks of acute otitis might not influence the child's development in any adverse way but persistent attacks might and Howie, Ploussard and Slayes (1975) found that babies who had one attack in the first year of life were more likely to have numerous further attacks in the first 6 years of life. It is very likely that acute otitis media may trigger chronic secretory otitis media which does have linguistic and educational sequelae.

Although it has been shown from the analysis of the Nottingham data that screening tests can be effective in detecting conductive hearing losses associated with otitis media even in babies (Haggard and Gannon, 1985), the fluctuating nature of this condition and the variable onset limit the effectiveness of any 'single event' screen in this respect. Clearly no method can detect a condition that has not yet become manifest and it must be appreciated that any screening programme will have limitations in this respect. There may be a need to introduce a certain degree of flexibility to test hearing at any time if there are suspicions that a hearing problem may have developed and this idea does not fit easily within a normal screening programme which, operationally, is timed according to the child's age.

The principal objective in any hearing screening programme is to identify cases likely to have hearing disorders of *medical and/or educational significance*. The criteria for assessing the significance of hearing problems will depend upon the focus of interest. Very few conditions affecting hearing are life threatening, with the possible exception of the rare state of cholesteatoma and the even rarer condition of childhood acoustic neuroma. Acute episodes of otitis media often respond well to medical treatment and may not necessarily have any educational or developmental significance. On the other hand chronic suppurative otitis media (CSOM), or glue ear, might be very significant from the developmental and educational point of view without qualifying for urgent treatment on medical grounds alone. In the case of sensori-neural hearing loss the major needs are for hearing aid and educational treatment rather than medical or surgical intervention (although surgery might offer some possibilities in a limited number of cases now that cochlea implants have become available).

Having established that the medical and educational significance of the hearing disorder is the primary guiding factor, a pathway of compromise must now be steered in order that a workable screening method can be devised. First, the question of whether we wish to screen for impairment, disability, or pathology must be answered. From the medical standpoint pathology may be of primary interest but the final decision as to whether action is required will usually be made on the basis of whether the resulting hearing disorder is likely to affect the child's health or general development. Ultimately it is the child's facility to hear speech that will to a very large extent determine the language growth and so a test of hearing for speech would seem to be a sensible choice. The very earliest hearing screening tests in 1924 did, in fact, utilise spoken numbers recorded on a phonograph. Children listened through headphones and had to write down the numbers they heard as the level of the words was gradually lowered. For various reasons to do with calibration and standardisation, speech tests were replaced in the late 1930s and early 1940s by pure tone tests following the advent of the pure tone audiometer. The pure tone audiometric type of test appeared to have more scientific sophistication and this may well be the reason why it has remained with us as the most commonly applied screening test for nearly half a century. It is important to realise, however, that while pure tone measurements record a level of impairment, such impairment may not necessarily be associated with a significant speech perception disability.

The dilemmas of hearing screening have been discussed by Haggard and Robinson (1986) and they argue that there should be a greater orientation towards auditory disability rather than impairment or pathology although they acknowledge the lack of relevant data on auditory disability. Until clearer guidelines have been established from well-conducted research of a higher quality than that hitherto available, the traditional hearing screening methods will no doubt prevail, and with some justification. There is, however, a need for those engaged in such work to analyse their techniques in depth, as described in this book. There is also a need for the objectives to be clearly defined according to Haggard and Robinson's classifications of pathology/impairment/disability distinctions.

THE BASIC REQUIREMENTS FOR A SCREENING TEST IN THE FIRST YEAR OF LIFE

When all the theoretically desirable aims and objectives have been defined we are left with the reality of what can be achieved in practice. Leaving aside the older pre-school child for the present and concentrating on babies in the first year of life, it is clearly not going to be possible to utilise tests of the understanding of speech. It is, however, possible to ensure that the baby responds to certain quiet levels of sounds and, furthermore, to check that sounds of different frequency content are heard.

The choice of a screening level

In the absence of special acoustically treated test rooms it is clearly not possible to test at threshold levels of hearing. Measurements of the acoustic characteristics of test environments in clinic locations in Nottinghamshire are discussed in Chapter 7 and these confirmed that most of the energy of the ambient noise is distributed in the low frequency region. Despite the recording of a fairly high ambient noise level of 35/40 dB overall it is, in fact, found that for frequencies above 1 kHz there is little in excess of 25 dB. There is some sense, therefore, in specifying that the stimulus levels to be used in free field testing in such environments should be 25–35 dB(A) and this indeed is what has happened in practice. Several practical constraints have dictated this level. First, most of the traditional sounds used over the years have either been produced mechanically or have been spoken in the live context by the tester and it is virtually impossible consistently to reproduce sounds at levels much quieter than 35 dB in such a situation. Secondly, there is some suggestion that babies' hearing threshold may be somewhat higher in the first months of life than that recorded for young adults. It is not clear whether this is a correct interpretation of the situation in the physiological sense or whether it is simply a question of needing a suprathreshold level before overt behavioural responses can be elicited.

Thus for a variety of reasons the minimum screening levels for use with babies in the first year of life are in the region of 25/35 dB.

The choice of test sounds and the analysis of frequency content

A hearing screening test will only meet its objective if the children or babies released from the net are the ones who hear speech well. Speech is complex in its acoustical make-up and no simple screening test can sample all of the complex features. It is, however, possible to go some way towards this objective by checking that the baby/child responds to the range of frequencies contained in normal speech. The objective is to ensure that a sample of low frequencies, middle frequencies and high frequencies can be heard. To achieve this it is not acceptable to present sounds of broad spectral component, that is sounds which contain many frequencies, because a response may occur only to a certain indefinable frequency range within the sound. Unfortunately, such sounds have been applied quite commonly and their use has resulted in cases with significant hearing loss being missed by the screening test.

In the condition known as high frequency hearing loss, the low and middle tones in speech may be heard at normal loudness but the affected child cannot hear the high frequencies. The effect for the child will be that although speech is heard due to the presence of the lower frequencies, it is not distinct because it lacks the higher frequencies. Some sounds may be entirely lacking and others will be

27

Table 2.2: Sounds of broad frequency spectra which are *not* suitable for hearing screening purposes

---

Stirring a cup with a spoon
Crinkling of tissue paper
Whispered and voiced speech
Forced 's' consonant
Watch tick
'ps' or 'ts' and 'tut' sounds
Baby rattles

---

distorted. This condition can seriously affect children in the formative years of speech and language growth and because the child responds to very quiet levels of sound, hearing lower frequency components, the condition is often overlooked with the resulting misdiagnosis of the nature of the child's speech and language problems. Table 2.2 lists sounds which are known to have indefinable broad-band frequency spectra and as such are not satisfactory for screening tests.

Sound spectrograms showing the distribution of energy in the speech frequency for some of these stimuli are given in Figures 2.1– 2.4. The analysis method used here, although rather limited for scientific scrutiny, gives a very clear pictorial representation of the content of the sound by displaying frequencies on the vertical (ordinate) scale and time on the horizontal (abscissa) scale. The relative intensities of the components are depicted by the depth of the shading. It can be seen that the sounds in question contain shading throughout the speech frequency range from 500 Hz up to 8 kHz and cannot, therefore, be used to check specific frequencies within this range. Analysis of the numerous brands of tissue paper shows a very similar broad frequency pattern and this may be somewhat surprising because subjectively the sound may appear to be high pitched. Similarly the forced 's' consonent may be thought to be high frequency but the spectrogram indicates components throughout the speech range, albeit with a fairly strong band in the high frequency region. If, however, a baby responded to this stimulus it is possible that the response may be occurring to any of the frequencies present. The broad band vertical bar on the 'cup and spoon' trace corresponds to the impact noise created when the spoon contacts the cup. As a general rule most sounds of impact nature display this abrupt onset and broad band frequency pattern. The spectrogram of the 'whisper' also demonstrates a wide frequency

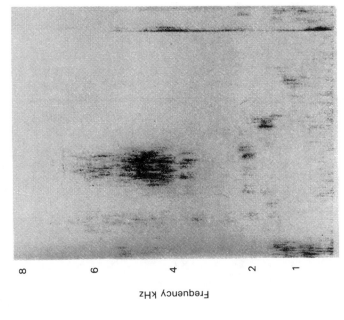

Figure 2.1: Spectogram of cup stirred with spoon

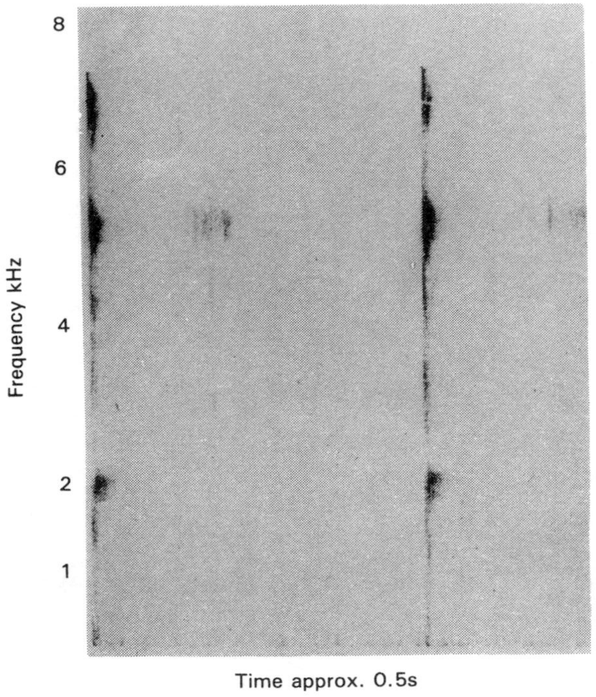

8
6
4
2
1
Frequency kHz
Time approx. 0.5s

Figure 2.2: Spectogram of whisper

8
6
4
2
1
Frequency kHz
Time approx. 0.5s

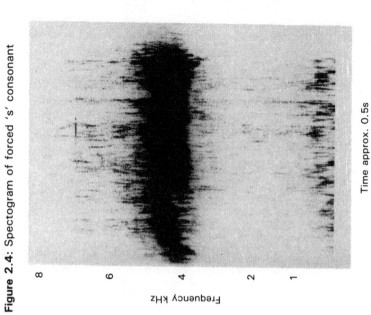

Figure 2.3: Spectogram of crinkled tissue paper

Time approx. 0.5s

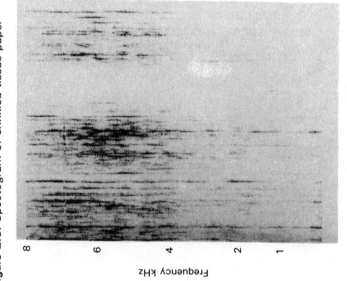

Figure 2.4: Spectogram of forced 's' consonant

Time approx. 0.5s

Table 2.3: Sounds with discrete frqeuency content which *are* suitable for hearing screening tests

High frequencies	Frequency range
Special high frequency rattle	Above 4 kHz (peak energy at > 10 kHz)
Very quiet 's' consonant	Approximately 4–5 kHz
Pure tones*	
Warble tones	Any frequency of choice
Narrow band noises	
Middle frequencies	
Pure tones*	
Warble tones	Any frequency of choice
Narrow band noises	
Low frequencies	
Quiet human 'hum'	Less than 500 Hz
Pures tones*	
Warble tones	Any frequency of choice
Narrow band noises	

*But not in a free field setting.

range which includes low frequencies. Devoicing does not remove low frequencies entirely.

In contrast to the wide range of sounds with broad band frequency spectra we have only a limited range of sounds with well-defined discrete frequency content and most of these are produced by electronic means. The list of acceptable sounds for hearing screening purposes is given in Table 2.3 and spectrograms of the acceptable 'conventional' screening sounds are given in Figures 2.5–2.7. Notice that the 's' consonant can produce a very discrete high frequency trace in the 4 kHz region if it is produced at a quiet level. The sound must not broaden into a 'sh' for this will produce a broad frequency trace. The high-frequency rattle shown in Figure 2.5 is the specially manufactured version available from the Department of Audiology, University of Manchester, and the peak energy for this is to be found in the region above 10 kHz. This is above the range of the spectrograms shown here and above the range of most simple sound level meters.

The 'minimal voice' trace shows a very good low frequency representation. The trace was, however, obtained from an

Figure 2.5: Spectogram of high frequency rattle

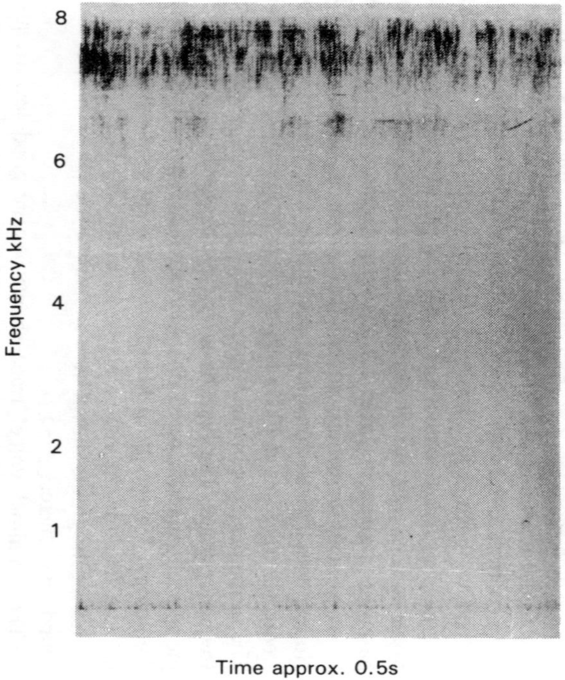
8
6
Frequency kHz
4
2
1
Time approx. 0.5s

Figure 2.6: Spectogram of 's' consonant

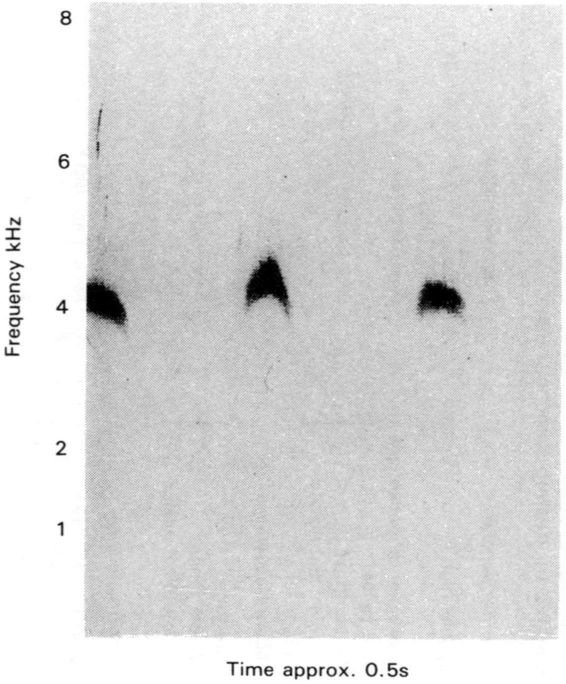
8
6
Frequency kHz
4
2
1
Time approx. 0.5s

Figure 2.7: Spectogram of minimal voice (hum)

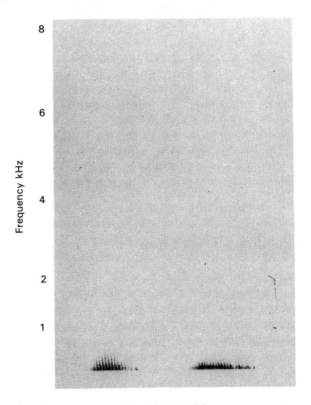

Time approx. 0.5s

experienced audiologist who had practised and analysed the sound. In a study reported by McCormick (1983) it was concluded that the use of a 'hum' stimulus was more reliable than 'minimal voice' in producing the low frequency characteristic. The 'hum' for the male or female does not extend beyond 500 Hz if produced at the necessary quiet level of 35 dB(A) needed for a hearing screening test.

The use of xylophones or chime bars of different centre frequency has been recommended by some audiologists and it is possible to produce sounds which are rich in certain frequencies if they are made with a soft striker. By their very design and tuneful

33

nature such sounds are, however, rich in harmonic content and it is difficult consistently to reproduce the desired frequency content at the correct screening level with such instruments.

To summarise the situation, in the absence of the facility of electronic noises, the only sounds recommended for hearing screening tests are the high frequency rattle, the consonant 's' and the 'hum'. This choice is determined by the discrete frequency content of these three sounds. The situation improves considerably if electronically generated sounds are used because these can be designed specifically to produce any frequency or frequency range of choice. The question now to be considered is whether babies respond to electronic sounds as well as they do to the more conventional sounds which have been used in the past for hearing screening purposes.

Babies responsiveness to test sounds

The literature has for many years been full of reference to terms such as the 'meaningfulness', 'biological significance', and 'effectiveness' of test sounds. It has been observed that babies respond more readily to certain sounds, for example, Froeschels and Beebe (1946), Eisenberg (1965), Ling, Ling and Doehring (1970) noted that pure tones were less effective than noise bands in evoking infant responses to sounds. Bender (1967) demonstrated that infants responded more readily to warble tones than to pure tones. Frequent reference is made in the literature to the meaningfulness of speech sounds and to the apparent abstract and artificial nature of electronic sounds. In the days prior to the widespread use of electronic equipment the pioneering work of Ewing and Ewing (1947) had established numerous general principles including: (a) that signals below 4 kHz evoke responses more easily than those above 4 kHz; and (b) that patterned sounds, particularly those in the speech — hearing range, are more effective stimuli than pure tones.

The explanation for what appears to be a consensus knowledge concerning the general idea of meaningfulness and responsiveness may depend heavily upon the acoustics of the sound as well as the nature and origin. Mendel (1968) showed that when the loudness and duration of stimuli were held constant, infants between the ages of 4 and 11 months were more responsive to broad-band spectrum sounds than to narrow-band spectrum sounds. The 'bandwidth' of the noise in question can be a significant factor. The more primitive sounds of percussion toys, rattles and speech all have broad frequency spectra relative to the more precisely definable electronic noises such as warble tones. Unfortunately, very few studies considered the effect of bandwidth on responsiveness and this has no doubt distorted the general conclusion about the 'meaningfulness' or 'appropriateness' of test sounds. The ideal experiment in which bandwidth is kept constant when comparing test sounds would be possible to perform but is probably not worth doing now in view of the known advantages of using frequency specific sounds (i.e. narrow bandwidth) to verify that babies are responsive at discrete and representative frequencies in the speech frequency range.

The evaluation of a warbler for hearing screening

In a questionnaire survey (McCormick, 1986) a warble tone screening instrument was evaluated in terms of the users' acceptance and satisfaction with the instrument and the general responsiveness of babies to such stimuli. A questionnaire was circulated to staff in all the known areas where a newly introduced 'meg' screening warbler (Figure 2.8) had been purchased. The replies included information from a total of 478 users of the instrument. In answer to the question 'In a distraction test do you find that babies are much less responsive, slightly less responsive, just as responsive, slightly more responsive, much more responsive, to the warble tones compared to other sounds?' the replies were as follows:

Much less responsive	9 per cent
Slightly less responsive	16 per cent
Just as responsive	44 per cent
Slightly more responsive	13 per cent
Much more responsive	18 per cent

Thus 75 per cent of the respondents found that babies were just as or more responsive to the warble sounds compared with the other sounds used in screening. In fact, the overall balance was slightly more favourable to the warble tones than to the other sounds. The other sounds used, some of which were acceptable in terms of frequency content and others not acceptable, included:

Figure 2.8: Warbler

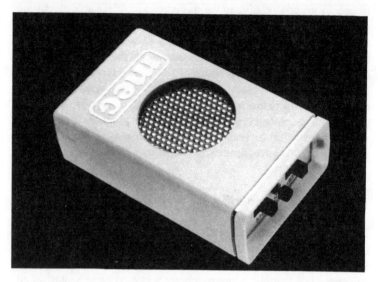

High frequency rattle used by 95 per cent of respondents
Consonant 's'   used by 59 per cent of respondents
'Hum'   used by 51 per cent of respondents
Voice   used by 38 per cent of respondents
Chime bars   used by 10 per cent of respondents
Cup and spoon   used by 8 per cent of respondents
Voiced 'oo' sound   used by 5 per cent of respondents
Tissue paper   used by 5 per cent of respondents
Whisper   used by 5 per cent of respondents

Other invalid and somewhat obscure items were also used, for example the rubbing and banging of wooden bricks and plucking the teeth of combs. It is rather curious and also disconcerting to see the appearance of such items in hearing screening tests.

The overall results from this survey confirmed that 94 per cent of the respondents were pleased with the use of the warble tones in the hearing screening context with babies. This was an interesting finding in view of the fact that 55 per cent of the respondents had no access to a sound-level meter to measure the level of the conventional sounds used in the screening test. In a previous study McCormick (1983) had found that the typical level produced by testers who had been trained to use sound-level meters, and had constant access to these instruments, was 40–50 dB rather than the specified level of less than 35 dB. It is likely that a large proportion of the respondents to the warbler survey were producing sound levels for the non-warble sounds at least 10 dB and in some cases 25 dB louder than the fixed levels on the warble tone instruments of 25 dB or 35 dB. Such an imbalance might well have produced a measure of responsiveness which did not favour the use of warble tones but this did not prove to be the case. The lesson to be learnt from these practical surveys is that comparative studies should equate the loudness of the stimuli in question. In reality it is not possible to quote a precise and repeatable level for human or mechanical sounds produced in a live context, for the variability is at least 5 dB or more for the same tester on any single test occasion and 10 dB or more for different testers and for different test occasions.

Warble tones and other electronic noises can be reproduced with a very high degree of uniformity and this is a great advantage. Not all electronic sounds are suitable for use in an open room setting and in particular pure tones fall into this category. Pure tones are only suitable for use with headphones rather than in an open space setting because of the phenomenon of standing waves which make such sounds susceptible to uncontrollable variation in the intensity level reaching the ears. The problem here is that of interference between the direct pressure wave emanating from the instrument's speaker, and reflected waves which travel a longer pathway. The resulting interference can introduce an intensity difference of 20 dB or so at the ear according to whether the direct and reflected waves have an additive or cancelling effect at the ear depending upon their relative phase. In view of this uncontrollable aspect of pure tone free field stimuli it is not recommended that such sounds be used in anything other than a headphone type of presentation. Warble tones have the advantage that they are not so susceptible to this standing wave effect and they also have a greater bandwidth which, as we have seen, is likely to produce greater responsiveness from the baby. The warble characteristic is also a feature likely to increase responsiveness. Narrow-band noises, that is noises containing a range of frequencies within a defined band, at equal loudness, are also usable in a free field context without the risk of a standing wave effect.

SUMMARY

The objective and basic requirements for a hearing screening test have been described and the factors which determine the choice of test sounds have been discussed. The introduction of electronic devices into the hearing screening field has opened up new possibilities for establishing uniformity and standardisation.

3

Utilising Parents' Suspicions: The Hints for Parents Approach

Numerous workers have demonstrated that parents' observations of their babies' reactions to sounds are generally very reliable indicators of the presence of hearing disorders (Latham and Haggard, 1980; Lilholdt, Courtois and Kortholm, 1980; Hitchings and Haggard, 1983).

A PILOT STUDY

The pilot work of Latham and Haggard (1980) formed a foundation for further developments of the parents' handout approach in Nottinghamshire and it will be described in some detail here. In their early work they utilised a simple list of pointers which described children's reactions to sounds in the first five years of life. This list was intended for distribution by health visitors and in order to assess its effectiveness the pilot study covered two matched health sectors one of which incorporated a distribution scheme for the handout while the other did not. Both health sectors, however, incorporated a standard interview between the health visitor and the parents in which questions about their baby's hearing were asked. The trial was incorporated into the normal work of the health visitor and each parent and child were seen twice over a period of between 1 and 6 months. At the beginning of each interview the parents were asked the question 'Do you think that your child is hearing normally?' The answers were noted and in one of the health sectors (the experimental sector) the clues' form was then given to the parents with the suggestion that it should be kept and the child's behaviour checked against it from time to time.

Over a 6-month period records were obtained on 780 children,

371 of which were in the experimental sector and 409 were in the control sector.

The analysis of the results of this study indicated more parental suspicion in the experimental sector but the numbers were too small to be statistically significant. The effectiveness of the parental questioning undertaken by the experimental and the control sectors was considered to be worthy of further investigation. The records showed that there had been an overall increase of 37.5 per cent in the number of babies/children referred to Medical Officers for hearing assessment during the trial period compared with the number in the corresponding period prior to the trial. It was concluded, therefore, that the mere act of posing the question about hearing prompted referrals for hearing assessment and that a more elaborately planned and controlled study was needed to isolate the additional contribution of the 'Clues' list distribution.

Of further interest from this study was the finding that only one parent out of 780 displayed active but unfounded concern about their offspring's hearing. Latham and Haggard commented:

> Considering that virtually all mothers of late-ascertained deaf children complain of the difficulty they have had in making professionals share their convictions that the child could not hear, our figures suggest that the 'Fussy Mother' is an irrelevant myth. So, where deafness is concerned, the supposed need to reassure the worrying parent should have no place in the education or in the taught professional lore of health visitors.

Further documented evidence of the value of parents' suspicions

Further investigations were undertaken in Nottinghamshire by Hitchings and Haggard (1983) to clarify issues not resolved within the early pilot study. In this case analysis of a more comprehensive set of data was undertaken to determine more information about the specificity and nature of the increased referrals.

The second investigation was designed to obtain evidence of the spread of the effect from the previous study to other children seen by the same health visitors in the affected districts, particularly in later months and years. For this purpose the two unaffected health districts in the authority served as control groups. The results confirmed that there had been a significant increase ($P < 0.001$) in the number of referrals for hearing assessment, in babies of less than 12 months of age, in the experimental groups but this increase was not evident in the control groups. There was also an increase in the number of babies under one year of age who were confirmed as having hearing impairment or needing surveillance and this effect was not apparent in the control groups. Thus increased referrals initiated by parental questioning led to earlier identification of hearing impairments in babies but did not result in loss of specificity.

The hints for parents 'Can your baby hear you?' form

Having obtained sufficient evidence to confirm that parental suspicion could be exploited in a systematic way by parental questioning the writer improved the original form of Latham and Haggard concentrating just on the first year of life. The form shown in Figure 3.1 was constructed and has been used routinely in Nottinghamshire since 1982. The form is given to parents by their health visitor during the first home visit and it is referred to again at the time of the routine distraction test screen which is performed when the baby is 6 to 7 months of age. Approximately 50,000 copies of the form have been issued to families in the Nottinghamshire area since it was introduced in the authority and only two or three cases of unnecessary referral have been recorded. This is taken as very strong evidence that the use of the form does not cause anxiety in the minds of parents whose babies hear well (that is to say the form has good specificity). It does, however, help to bring to the attention of the clinicians those babies who have hearing problems (good sensitivity). It has not been possible to obtain precise sensitivity and specificity ratings for the form as an isolated part of the community care because this is now only one of a number of new initiatives being assessed simultaneously in the authority. The use of the form can, however, be justified purely on the grounds that it provides a reference from which suspicion or satisfaction about a baby's reactions to sound can be gauged, and it does this simply and economically within an existing health care system. The 'hints for parents' approach serves as a valuable adjunct and safety catch net for use alongside other screening methods. A particular virtue is that it utilises long-term observations rather than single one-off assessments of the type used in community screening programmes. The significance of this virtue should not be underestimated for a

41

Figure 3.1: Hints for parents

"Can your baby hear you?"

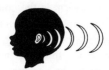

Here is a checklist of some of the general signs you can look for in your baby's first year:-

YES/NO

Shortly after birth
Your baby should be startled by a sudden loud noise such as a hand clap or a door slamming and should blink or open his eyes widely to such sounds.

By 1 Month
Your baby should be beginning to notice sudden prolonged sounds like the noise of a vacuum cleaner and he should pause and listen to them when they begin.

By 4 Months
He should quieten or smile to the sound of your voice even when he cannot see you. He may also turn his head or eyes toward you if you come up from behind and speak to him from the side.

By 7 Months
He should turn immediately to your voice across the room or to very quiet noises made on each side if he is not too occupied with other things.

By 9 Months
He should listen attentively to familiar everyday sounds and search for very quiet sounds made out of sight. He should also show pleasure in babbling loudly and tunefully.

By 12 Months
He should show some response to his own name and to other familiar words. He may also respond when you say 'no' and 'bye bye' even when he cannot see any accompanying gesture.

> Your health visitor will perform a routine hearing screening test on your baby between seven and nine months of age. She will be able to help and advise you at any time before or after this test if you are concerned about your baby and his development. If you suspect that your baby is not hearing normally, either because you cannot answer yes to the items above or for some other reason, then seek advice from your health visitor.

©
Produced by Dr. Barry McCormick
Children's Hearing Assessment Centre, General Hospital, Nottingham NG1 6HA

condition such as hearing impairment which may fluctuate, may be progressive, or may be of sudden and sometimes unpredictable onset.

Despite its attractions this approach cannot be used in isolation as a definitive screening method for the following reasons:

1. It is insensitive to hearing problems affecting selective frequencies only (for example high tone hearing loss).
2. It may not necessarily help to identify babies with partial hearing problems with associated abnormal loudness function who may not hear quiet sounds but can hear louder sounds at normal subjective loudness levels, and
3. Not all parents can be reached by the method either because of reading or language difficulties or because of poor motivation or complacency.

SUMMARY

Parents' suspicions of the presence of hearing impairment in their off-spring are known to be reliable and should be used as routine indicators in screening programmes. The issue of a form of the 'hints for parents' type described in this chapter offers the simplest and most convenient system for unifying this approach.

4

The Modified Distraction Test for Babies between Six Months and Eighteen Months

The distraction (or distracting) test was first described by Ewing and Ewing in 1944 and it is now the most commonly used routine hearing screening test for babies. The test is based on the principle that babies turn to locate sounds presented on the horizontal plane through the ears if the sounds have sufficient novelty and if the attention state is suitable adjusted. Two testers are required to undertake the test. One presents the sound stimuli out of visual field and the other captures and then controls the baby's attention in the forward direction (see Figure 4.1).

Despite the fact that this test has been adopted in one form or another for 40 years or so, its general record of success in the screening context has been very poor. The test has been justly criticised for delaying access to help for many deaf babies because false reassurance has been given to parents about their baby's hearing status on the basis of findings from invalid test technique. A number of studies undertaken in recent years have raised serious doubts about the reliability of the test and the consistent finding to emerge from these studies is that fewer than 10-20 per cent of congenitally deaf children are detected by the method (DHSS, 1981); National Deaf Children's Society, 1983; Martin and Moore, 1979; McCormick, 1983). This is an appalling state of affairs for a test which is applied to nearly every child. A report of a survey undertaken by the Health Visitors' Association (1977) confirmed that all infants were screened in their first year of life in the 198 health districts from which usable replies were received.

It seems logical to conclude from these findings that the test, as generally applied. has thoroughly wasted time and resource. The fact that its applications has resulted in delayed access to help, and the giving of false reassurance, raises the issue of whether the cost

Figure 4.1: Distraction test situation

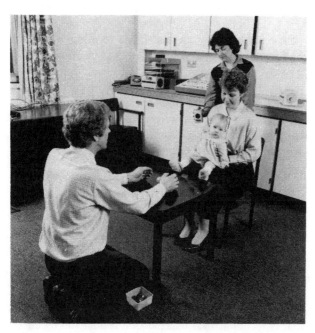

and resource needed to maintain a distraction test screening programme can be justified. There is a need to question the evidence for continuing with the method in community health care settings. The economics of the test are such that it requires expenditure of only a few pounds per test per child but a few million pounds each year for coverage throughout the UK. Analysing the figures according to the cost per child detected we arrive at a figure of several thousand pounds for each congenitally deaf child detected or several hundred pounds for each child with a conductive loss.

The historical problems of this test have been considered by the author within the context of a local authority screening service and following detailed analysis of the test technique the factors which contributed to the poor reliability of the test have been isolated. With the incorporation of the improved test technique, to be outlined in this chapter, the success of the test in detecting hearing-impaired babies has improved substantially. The records showed that the service in question detected less than 20 per cent of deaf children in their first year of life prior to the incorporation of the improved techniques, and following their incorporation well over 70 per cent of the congenitally deaf babies were detected within their first year of life.

The main reasons why the test failed to achieve a satisfactory level of acceptability included such factors as insufficient care being taken to exclude visual clues from the test situation, the use of inadequate test sounds, and poor control over the baby's attention state prior to and during sound stimulus presentation. The situation reflected the inadequacies of the original training course and there is an urgent need for training-course content to be improved according to the guidelines presented in this chapter.

THE REQUIREMENTS FOR A GOOD DISTRACTION TEST

Age

To perform this test adequately in a screening context a baby must have matured to the stage of being able to sit erect and perform head turns in the horizontal plane. The test technique to be described is suitable for babies from 6 months of age up to approximately 18 months. It is recommended that the first test should be undertaken at 6 or 7 months and certainly no later than 8 months to minimise the delay in providing help for those babies affected by severe or profound hearing disorders. With some babies allowance may have to be made for prematurity but if doubt has been expressed about a baby's hearing it should be tested if possible or referred for diagnostic testing if screening is not possible. There are two good reasons for making this statement: first, there is a much higher incidence of sensori-neural hearing loss in premature babies (approximately ten times greater incidence than in full-term babies) and secondly, some premature babies are quite ready for the test at 7 or 8 months. If it transpires that the baby is developmentally not ready for the test the very fact that interest is being focused on hearing may prompt parents to express any concerns. Parental suspicion is known to be an extremely reliable indicator of the presence of hearing disorders in their offspring (see Chapter 3).

The distraction test is often used also for babies above the age of 18 months to complement other techniques and the modifications needed for older children will be discussed later.

Space

A quiet room (minimum 4 m × 4 m), with a calm relaxed atmosphere is required. The background (ambient) noise level should normally not exceed 35/40 dB(A) (see Chapter 7).

Personnel

Two trained testers *must* be available to administer the test.

Equipment

1. Low (coffee) table.
2. Selection of frequency specific sounds covering low, middle, and high speech frequencies, e.g. high frequency rattle, warble tones of different frequencies.
3. Sound-level indicator or meter (desirable although not essential if electronic warblers are used).

Organisation of the test situation

The baby should be seated on the parent's knee facing forward and sitting erect as shown in Figure 4.1. The parent must be instructed not to react in any way when sounds are presented, for even the slightest movements on their part could initiate a response from the child and thereby invalidate the test. The testers should observe carefully for any such behaviour during the actual test.

One tester works at the front, preferably kneeling down behind the low table facing the child. This tester's role is to capture and then control the child's attention to just the right degree so that at the appropriate time, when the sound stimulus is presented, the baby is suitably freed from auditory, visual, and tactile distractions. The function of the second worker is to remain outside the child's vision completely divorced from the baby's attention ready to present each sound stimulus at the appropriate location and time.

Let us consider the testers' roles in full detail.

The worker at the front

This person is responsible for directing the test and to do this to full effect it may be necessary for him/her to speak to the second tester. Although this is permissible it is vitally important that he/she does not look at the partner or give any clue to indicate that there is anyone behind the child. The cue for the sound stimulus to be inserted should be the phasing out of the activity being used to capture and control the baby's attention. The activity should be simple, e.g. spinning a small object on the low table to bring the attention to a peak and then phasing the attention by covering the object with the hands. If the baby's attention starts to drift it can be re-captured and manipulated simply by moving a finger or gently tapping the object on the table whilst keeping it concealed under the hands. The aim should be to keep the baby's attention on the table surface rather than on the tester. The sequence is shown in Figure 4.2 (i–vi). This technique has the advantage that it enables the tester to observe the baby's eyes without any danger of forming eye contact, or eye fixation, which could over-captivate the baby's attention. The requirement for good distraction is to keep the activity very simple and calm rather than indulge in gross and complex behaviour.

Examples of poor distraction procedures

Cluttered display. A table littered with other toys would be most unsuitable for the test. The table surface should be kept completely clear apart from the item being used for the attention capture.

Gross activity. A method often used, but not favoured by the author, is that of standing in front of the baby with a cuddly toy or a ball which is then quickly transferred to behind the distractor. This activity does not permit the necessary fine degree of control to be exercised over the baby's attention and the child often forms eye contact with the tester. A method commonly used for releasing this eye contact is for the distractor to look down at the floor, but in so doing the tester is no longer able to observe the nature of the baby's response or lack of response. The worker at the front is the only person in the room who can gauge the significance of any head-turn response according to the observed attention state and it is very poor practice not to observe the baby's face and specifically the eyes. It will be appreciated that the table surface technique

Figure 4.2: (i) Attention capture

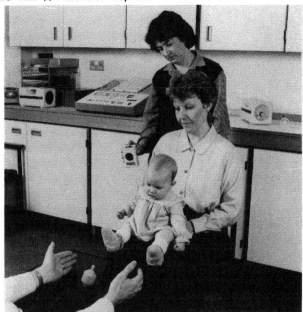

Figure 4.2: (ii) Phasing of attention

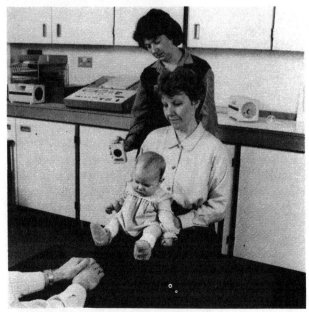

Figure 4.2: (iii) Fine manipulation of attention

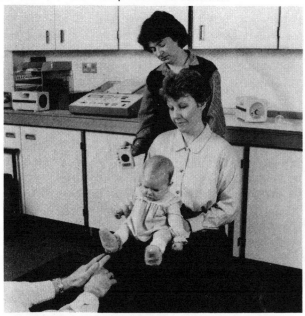

Figure 4.2: (iv) Head turn response

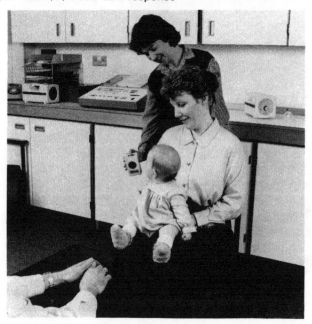

Figure 4.2: (v) Response reward

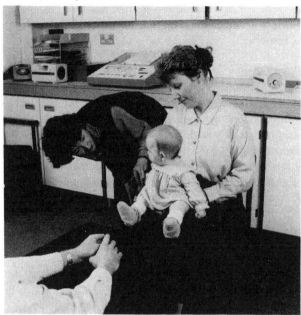

Figure 4.2: (vi) Attention brought forward

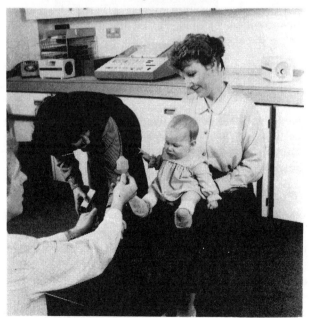

has considerable merit here and, in particular, the phasing of the activity with the hands followed by fine attention manipulating by slight finger movement leaves the distractor free to observe the baby's response.

Signalling location of sound source. It has already been stated that the distractor should not glance at the partner but equally there should be no other 'give away' signal such as the slightest gesture in the direction of the partner. This and many other suggestions presented here may seem to be obvious, but the writer has observed distractors pointing in the direction of the sound and when asked to justify this technique the testers advised that they had been trained to give a signal for the sound insertion and the point constituted the signal!

Poor timing. A very common error in the administration of the distraction test is that of over captivating the baby's attention without including suitably timed attention phases. The attention should be phased, by covering the item on the table with the hands, within a second or two of the maximum attention capture and then the fine finger manipulation should be continued for at least a further 5 or 10 seconds if the baby does not turn to locate the stimulus sound. Premature attention recapture without sufficient allocation of time for response will only prolong the test time and may lead to an abandonment of the test.

The worker at the rear

Although this worker does not direct the test the validity of the test depends to a very late degree upon his/her skill in presenting the *right sounds* at the *right place* at the *right time* (the three r's of the distraction test).

The right place

The sound source should be located on a horizontal level with the baby's ear at a distance of approximately one metre (or at a specified distance if warblers are used) from the ear outside the baby's field of vision (see Figure 4.3). A good reference position for locating the sound is in the vertical plane of the back of the chair in which the mother/father is seated with the baby, at arm's length from the corner of the chair and with the sound in the horizontal plane which passes

Figure 4.3: Correct location of sound stimulus

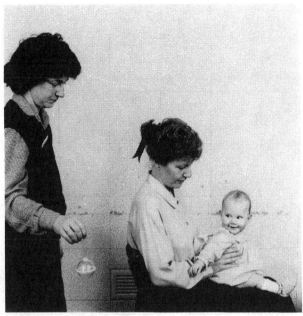

through the baby's ears. Nothing should be allowed to enter into the child's peripheral visual field including the sound source, the tester's shoe, hair shadows, etc. and it must be assumed that anything situated in front of the chair-back could be within the baby's peripheral vision.

Visual cueing is probably the most common invalidator of the distraction test and unless due care is taken to remove such cues the test will be of no value whatsoever. In setting up the test situation, prior to bringing in the baby, the tester must select a position in the room where there are no shadows cast in the forward direction by the worker at the back (Figure 4.4). Control may have to be effected on such shadows by switching off sets of lights, drawing certain curtains or blinds and positioning the parent's chair to achieve the optimum control, remembering that any change of lighting, for example if the sun starts to shine, might require adjustment. The tester should move to the test positions on each side to ensure not only that shadows are not present but also that there are no creaking floorboards, clothes rustling, shoe squeaks (or their footstep noises), or clinking jewellery.

Figure 4.4: Unacceptable shadow

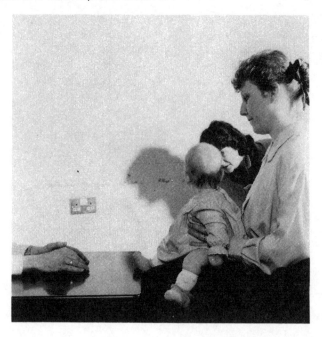

Having chosen the optimum position for excluding shadows it should then be checked for the presence of any reflections which may be detected by the baby from, for example, television screens, sterilisers, mirrors, or windows. Sources of such reflections should be covered, angled to different positions, or removed.

It is vital, of course, that the worker at the back does not talk to the distractor for this will immediately alert the baby to his/her presence and location. Also perfumes or aftershaves should not be worn for these may give olfactory cues.

The right time

The stimulus sound should be presented no longer than one second after the distractor covers the object at the front. If the baby does not respond immediately the stimulus should be presented for between 5 and 10 seconds whilst the distractor continues with the fine attention manipulation. The sound should not be 'rehearsed' before test presentation for this will lessen the possibility of obtaining a response later due to the loss of novelty or change in the sound environment.

54

The right sound

Only minimal levels (< 35 dB(A)) of sound are acceptable for a screening test and ideally a sound-level meter should be available so that the levels can be checked at intervals. A description of sound-level meters is given in Chapter 7.

It is necessary to test the baby's response to high and low frequencies in the speech frequency range. Briefly, if electronic warblers are not available, only the following sounds should be used unless the full frequency analysis of any alternative sounds can verify their validity:

High frequencies.

1. Special Manchester high frequency rattle shown in Figure 4.5 (centre frequency above 10 kHz).
2. Consonant 's' (approximately 4.5 kHz) repeated rhythmically. It must be a clear 's' and not 'sh' as the latter contains a wide band of frequencies.

Low frequencies. In the absence of electronic noises the only satisfactory low frequency sound for screening purposes is the 'hum' (less than 500 Hz). Rhythmical repetition of a nursery rhyme is all that is required. The frequency of the male or female produced 'hum' presented at minimal levels does not rise above 500 Hz regardless of the actual tune. Whispering and quiet speaking will invalidate the test because these sounds contain a wide range of frequencies.

Arousal items

The crinkling of tissue paper and gentle stirring of a spoon in a cup have been used in the past as test items but it is known that these are non-specific in their frequency content and it is not recommended that they be used. The justification for retaining them in the test has been that babies are reported to be particularly responsive to them and they may arouse a baby who is otherwise unresponsive. The disadvantage of indeterminate frequency content overshadows any potential advantage of such sounds.

55

Figure 4.5: Manchester high frequency rattle

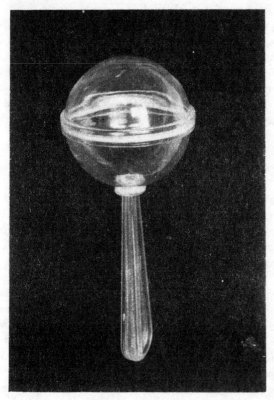

Electronic sounds — warblers

If an electronic device such as the 'meg' warbler is available this will produce the correct level of sound at select frequencies in the speech range and hence replace the need for the above 'conventional' sounds. The introduction of such technology is well received by parents.

The warble tone frequencies recommended as a minimum requirement are 500 Hz, 2 kHz and 4 kHz and a baby can pass the screening test by responding to each of these frequencies on each side. The 2 kHz tests the middle speech frequency range thus adding a useful addition to the distraction test. The manufacturer's instructions should be followed carefully, taking particular note of the settings and distance. The warblers must, of course, be held out of the field

Figure 4.6: Correct location of warbler (50 cm from the ear)

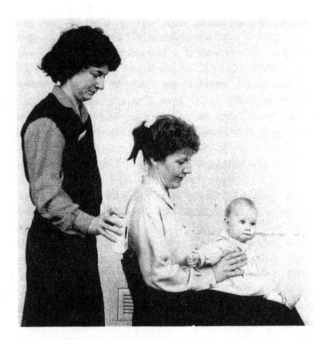

of vision. The ideal position for the device is 50 cm from the ear at an angle of 45° set back from the ear and this is shown in Figure 4.6.

A 25 dB or 30 dB setting is recommended in preference to the 35 dB or 40 dB settings and these lower settings are suitable in most routine test environments. It is, of course, vital that the interrupter switch is operated without any audible click.

Even if warblers are available it is still advisable for testers to retain their skills and practice with the 's', the rattle, and the 'hum' for these extend the range of sounds if a baby shows signs of boredom or habituation. The rattle does, of course, present a very high frequency sound thus giving additional information as a bonus, although it is by no means essential to check such high frequencies in a screening test if it can be shown that a baby responds well at 4 kHz.

It is recommended that, if available, warblers are used first during a test, and then the 's', 'hum' and rattle should be introduced if, for any reason, the baby is unresponsive and a more varied range of sounds is needed.

57

Criteria for passing the test

In the screening context, the only response from the baby that will constitute a pass is a definite and full 90° head turn in the direction of the sounds when presented at the minimal level. Low and high frequency sounds should be responded to in this way, and also the middle 2 kHz tone if warblers are available. If a baby consistently fails to respond to one sound, even if only on one side, then he/she should fail the screen and appropriate follow-up arrangements should be made. Eye glances in the direction of the sound or other possible signs of response cannot be accepted in the screening context. Even at the diagnostic level, skilled and experienced testers interpret these signs with great caution. The normal response for a baby at this age is a full head turn to locate the sound and if the baby does not show this behaviour there must be a reason worthy of investigation.

There may be a reason not related to hearing, which prevents the child from responding; it may be that the child is developmentally not ready for the test, the child may not be in a suitable state on the day, or the child may have some mental or physical disability. Such behaviour patterns need to be investigated outside the context of a screening test. The physical maturation of the baby to turn its head in the horizontal plane should be checked at the commencement of the test by focusing his/her visual gaze on, for example, a rattle and then checking to see if he/she will visually follow the items through a 90° arc to each side (see Figure 4.7). If the baby does not do this the distraction test will not be appropriate as a hearing screening test and if there are suspicions about the hearing this should be tested by experts using other methods.

To pass the screening test, combinations of responses to high and low frequency stimuli could be accepted, that is warble and conventional sound, on condition that the conventional sounds are presented at the correct screening level of less than 35 dB(A). In the situation when a baby does not appear to respond to the warble tones it is very easy to make the mistake of raising the level of the conventional sounds, perhaps subconsciously, thereby eliciting responses from some babies. The level of the conventional sounds should be checked very carefully with a sound-level meter in such circumstances.

A sample record form for documenting the screening test result is shown in Table 4.1. It can be seen that in this case the baby responded to all of the stimuli. In the absence of warble tone stimuli

Figure 4.7: Checking head turning ability with visual tracking

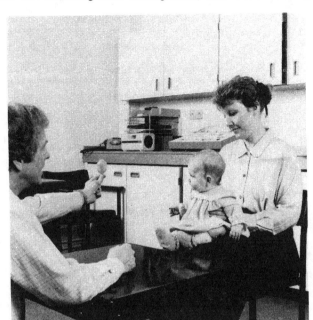

ticks would be required in the 'hum', 's', and rattle boxes, and it would be wise to have a double check on the 'hum' (this being the only sound outside the high frequency range). The results would be recorded as in Table 4.2 if warblers are not available and as in Table 4.3 if warble tone stimuli only are to be used for the screening test.

The final choice of screening criteria and record form must be left to local policy makers but the author recommends the use of the first record form completing the middle warble tone section first and only using the 'hum', 's', and 'rattle' sections if, for some reason, the baby does not appear to be responsive to the warble tones.

The consideration of the number of trials to be administered for each stimulus is complicated by attention drifts and uncontrollable distractions from extraneous noise. In the ideal situation the baby should respond to every stimulus presented at the screening level. If a response is not obtained at the quiet level but can be elicited at a raised level the indication could be that a hearing problem is present but another possibility is that the baby's attention might have drifted. A measure of consistency is needed here and if immediate

Table 4.1: Sample record form for the distraction test

	FREQUENCY					
	Low		Middle		High	
	hum	500 Hz	2 kHz	4 kHz	's'	H.F. rattle
Right ear	✔	✔	✔	✔	✔	✔
Left ear	✔	✔	✔	✔	✔	✔
		WARBLE TONES				

Table 4.2: Basic record form (no warbler)

	FREQUENCY			
	Low		High	
	hum	hum	's'	H.F. rattle
Right ear	✔	✔	✔	✔
Left ear	✔	✔	✔	✔

Table 4.3: Basic record form for warbler responses

	FREQUENCY		
	Low	Middle	High
	500 Hz	2 kHz	4 kHz
Right ear	✔	✔	✔
Left ear	✔	✔	✔
		WARBLE TONES	

60

responses are not obtained at the screening level the response must be obtained from two out of three presentations at the screening level to be acceptable.

IMPORTANT ADDITIONAL NOTES

Response reinforcement

Once the baby has turned to a particular sound the tester should reward the response by simple means such as a smile, vocal praise, or a tickle on the arm etc, and then he/she should stay in position until the distractor has regained the attention in the forward direction. Once the attention is off the tester he/she should then either stay on that side or move to the other side in an unpredictable sequence so that the baby cannot anticipate the side of presentation of subsequent stimuli.

No sound trials

It is important that the child's checking or searching behaviour should be observed and controlled for carefully during the test. This should be done by introducing 'no sound' trials in which the distractor captures, controls, and phases the attention in the normal way and the other tester moves in position as if to present a sound, but without actually presenting the sound. Ideally the number of 'no sound' trials should equal the number of 'sound' trials but in practice this may extend the test beyond the baby's optimum attention span. 'No sound' trials should, however, be used in every test situation at different stages during the test for this provides the only measure of checking or searching behaviour and, in addition, provides a safeguard for detecting the presence of any inadvertent and unwanted auditory, visual, or tactile cues. If a baby is observed to be checking it will certainly be necessary to include as many 'no sound' trials as 'sound' trials. It must be remembered that there is a high probability that the baby will turn to one side or the other even if no sounds are present. The objective within the test is to defeat this behaviour as far as possible by correct manipulation of attention in the forward direction without, of course, over captivating the attention.

Increasing the responsiveness

If a baby shows apparently no interest in a particular sound it might be useful for the distractor momentarily to incorporate the same sound in the activity at the front before phasing the attention. This is particularly useful when testing older children. Posing the question 'where is the noise?' may elicit a response in an otherwise unresponsive baby. If this technique is used it is vital that 'no sound' trials are also used with inclusion of 'where is the noise?' or 'find the noise' during these trials.

Introducing novelty

Babies beyond the age of 10 months may soon lose interest in the test sounds. They may turn once to satisfy their curiosity and then show little interest if the sounds are presented again. In such a situation it may be helpful to vary the order of presentation of the sounds to heighten novelty and in addition, match the sounds as described above.

Sound presentation interval

If the baby does not respond within 5 or 10 seconds it is unlikely that the attention will still be controlled to an optimum degree and the attention-gain activity should be introduced again by the distractor.

Observers

If other relatives or observers are in the room during the test they should be seated directly behind the distractor (i.e. in front of the baby) and as far away as possible. They should be instructed not to look at the person working behind the child at any time during the test. The distractor will be able to detect if the baby is searching for, or distracted by, the presence of such observers and if this proves to be a problem the observers must be asked to leave the room until the test is completed. If the technique of keeping the baby's attention on the table surface is applied correctly the presence of observers seated behind the distractor rarely poses problems and the distractor can see quite clearly if the baby is looking in the direction of the observer. It is very poor practice to seat observers to the side of or behind the baby because this is highly likely to initiate head turn towards that person, particularly if it is a member of the family. These localising responses may be misinterpreted as response to sound stimuli. It must be remembered that even in the absence of no sound stimuli there is a high probability that the baby will turn to one side or the other and the presence of a person to the side or behind will heighten this probability and reduce the reliability of the test. By seating the observer centrally in front of the baby there will be no tendency for that person's presence to initiate a head turn response to the side.

The need to include 'no sound' trials routinely in all test situations cannot be over-emphasised and if other observers are in the room the need is, of course, even greater.

If very young brothers or sisters are present during the test the most appropriate place for them to sit is hidden away immediately behind the mother's chair. A useful technique here is to tempt the child with a game of trains or buses with Mummy/Daddy in the front seat and they can sit in the back seat. They can be encouraged to hold tightly onto the steering wheel (i.e. the back of the parent's chair) and not to let go. The advantage of this method is that the tester at the back can keep control over the child ensuring that he/she does not give any clue, and the child can remain out of the baby's attention. The technique of placing the child in front is not recommended for very small children because they usually need the security of being next to their parents and even if they can be tempted to be some distance away they may not sit still or they may give clues to the baby.

If the technique of sitting behind the parent does not work and no other helpers are available to occupy the child in another room it may be necessary to seat the child on one side of the mother, test the ear on the opposite side, and then change sides. This is not, however, very satisfactory and there is a high chance that there will be difficulties with the child peering round to see the test sounds thereby invalidating the test.

SUMMARY

The distraction test is very simple in principle but there are many pitfalls which, unless avoided, can invalidate the test. These have been discussed in detail in this chapter and the requirements for a valid test have been presented based on the use of the warble tones either used alone or in combination with the more conventional screening sounds.

5

Testing the Hearing of Children with Mental Ages between Eighteen Months and Two-and-a-Half Years

By the time a child has reached a mental age of 18 months he/she should be able to understand simple verbal instructions. This broadens the horizon for hearing screen beyond the confines of auditory detection into the very important areas of auditory discrimination of speech. This age group is, beyond doubt, the most difficult and challenging for the hearing screener. The typical 18-month-old child may cry a lot and want to do the opposite of what adults request or desire. The child's normal negativisms and short variable attention span may challenge the skills of the tester to the full. The screening tests, whilst very simple in theory, may be difficult to apply in practice owing to the child's lack of co-operation. The tests to be described here are based on play methods, some of which were first described by Ewing and Ewing (1947) under the title of 'The Co-operative Test' (a term with intrinsic appeal to the sense of humour).

It is recommended that the screening test should be divided into two sections for this age group; (a) screening auditory discrimination, and (b) screening auditory acuity.

AUDITORY DISCRIMINATION

The objective here is to check that the child can hear and discriminate between simple speech instructions at very quiet listening levels. The task is one of auditory discrimination between speech sounds, rather than simple detection of a signal, and the minimum level of voice to be used in the test is 40 dB(A) (that is 5 dB higher than the pass criteria level for the detection of sound in the distraction test). It is strongly recommended that the voice level should be checked using a sound-level meter or speech-level indicator whenever these tests are performed (see Chapter 7 for a description of these instruments). In the absence of such instruments the voice level should be gauged prior to the test by checking that an adult with normal hearing can just hear a faint signal but not decipher the intelligibility of the words when listening at a distance of 3 metres. This level of voice should then be used at a distance of 1 metre from the child.

It is important to understand that the test is designed to screen the child's ability to understand quiet levels of speech which include voicing and not whispered signals. Whispering distorts speech because of the removal of voicing cues and it does not, therefore, constitute typical speech in which the relationships between the different vowel, consonant, and dipthong sound are conserved.

Another important condition for this test is that the child should not be permitted to observe the speaker's face because he/she might detect visual speech clues (that is lipread or speech read the articulatory movements of speech). If the test is performed facing the child the lower half of the speaker's face should be well covered with a hand or a piece of paper and the same technique should be used at any time if the child glances in the direction of the tester.

Speech materials

A variety of speech materials can be used depending upon the testers' personal preference and the child's interests and abilities. The following are presented as alternatives.

The four-toy eyepointing test (McCormick)

This technique offers the simplest possible version of a speech discrimination test requiring the minimum degree of co-operation from the child. Two pairs of items from the McCormick toy discrimination test (described in Chapter 6) are used, namely a cup and duck and a spoon and shoe. With the child seated on his/her parent's knee facing the tester the items are brought out individually and a check is made with the parent that each toy is known to the child. The items are displayed in an arc on a table situated between the child and the tester, allowing at least 20 cm separation between each toy as in Figure 5.1. At a normal conversational level of voice the tester then asks, for example, 'Where is the shoe?'. The minimum acceptable response from the child should be a gaze in the direction of that item with a clear visual fixation on the item. If no response is

Figure 5.1: Four toy eyepointing test situation

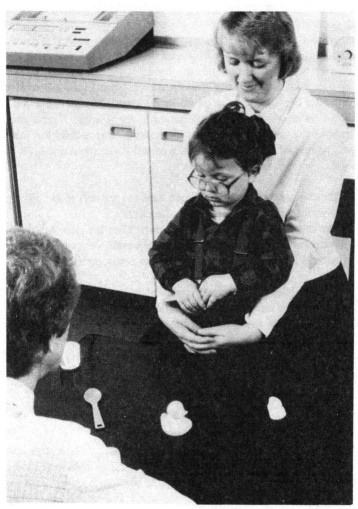

recorded the instruction should be changed to 'Look at the shoe'. Correct responses should be rewarded with, for example, a smile, a hand clap, or other form of praise. Following two or three trials at a conversational level, the voice level should then be lowered to the minimal 40 dB(A) level and the face should be covered to obliterate lip-reading clues. With only four items in the display there is clearly a high possibility of chance response or a learning effect if the toys are requested in a set order and this must be avoided. To increase the validity of the test the toys could be given an occasional shuffle in their position in the display; this also helps to recapture any drifts in the child's attention particularly if it is done in a lively manner. The child passes this part of the screening test if he/she consistently identifies the correct items at the minimal level of voice with a score of at least four correct responses out of five (or 80 per cent) requests at the 40 dB(A) level. Obvious drifts in the child's attention should be discounted in the scoring. Eyepointing involves the minimum possible co-operation from a child but there are certain pitfalls which must be avoided if the technique is to be valid:

1. There must be a clear separation between the toys in the display to avoid ambiguity in the gaze direction.
2. The response should be recorded only when the gaze has fixed. Premature rewarding of a response as a child's eyes sweep in the general direction of the stimulus item could invalidate the test.

If the child is mature enough and will co-operate by finger pointing to the items then it may be possible to apply the test on each side rather than from the front. In this case the tester should position him/herself at a distance of one metre at right angles to the ear obtaining consistent (80 per cent correct) responses on each side.

The results can then be recorded as 'pass' or 'refer for further testing' for each ear rather than for the binaural condition from the front.

The co-operative test

The following is an account of the traditional co-operative test technique, the basic principle of which was first described by the Ewings. It can be a very satisfying test to perform with the more co-operative child but it does require more skill and more time to apply than the four-toy eyepointing test.

The objective is to develop a 'giving' game and to achieve maximum sensitivity the items chosen should be acoustically very similar. A test using mummy, teddy, and dolly, will clearly be more challenging and sensitive than a test using mummy, boat, and table. Apart from the rather gross acoustic phenomic differences in the latter selection the number of syllables also give large clues to the identity of the items. Thus to increase the sensitivity of the test the items should have the same number of syllables and they should have

Figure 5.2: The co-operative test

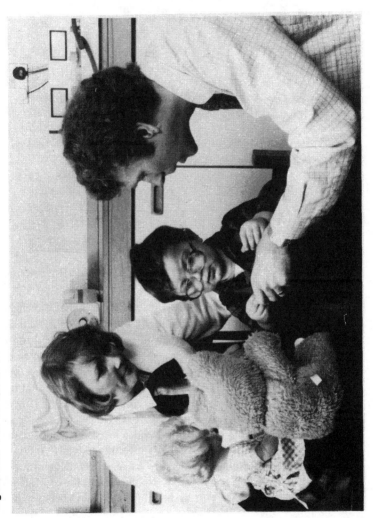

Figure 5.3: Guided response

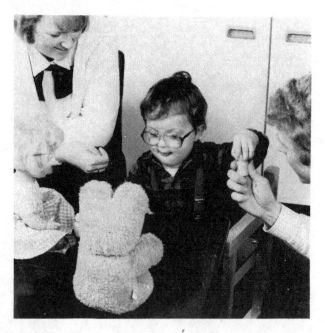

certain acoustic similarities. The writer's preferred choice of items are mummy (or daddy), teddy and dolly (or baby). Other suitable choices might include doll, dog, ball, or cup, duck, dog and so on.

The test starts with the child seated on his/her parent's knee or, if willing, on a chair adjacent to the parent. Each item is then brought out and a check is made with the parent to ensure that it is known to the child. The items are spaced out on the table (Figure 5.2) and then in a conversational level of voice the tester demonstrates the giving game using wooden bricks or other suitable objects. The statement might be 'Let's give this to teddy' followed by the tester performing the action. After a few demonstration responses by the tester, and possibly also the parent, the child should then be prompted to take part by holding a brick and being guided by the tester when the instruction is given (for example 'Give this one to dolly'). It might be wise to place the brick in the child's hand and then hold the child's hand to guide the first few responses as shown in Figure 5.3. This guiding method has the advantage of restraining the child and avoiding impulsive responses based on the

Figure 5.4: Correct position for the co-operative test

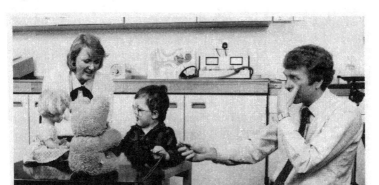

child's preference rather than the tester's instruction. By gradually releasing the hold of the child's hand the tester can determine whether the child is attempting to respond impulsively or whether he/she is conditioned and waiting for the next instruction. If the child is still not showing restraint more examples of guided response should be included.

Once the correct degree of conditioning has been achieved the tester should lower the voice level to 40 dB(A) and present the instructions in varying order, perhaps occasionally perserverating on one item if the child shows a tendency to respond in a set sequence. The choice of item for each instruction should be quite casual and hence unpredictable. The test should be performed at a distance of 1 metre from each ear and at right angles to the ear (Figure 5.4) ensuring consistency of responses at the minimal listening level without visual clues.

Another option

If a child will not perform with either of the above methods it is worth trying a familiar technique using the following requests: 'Show me your hair', 'Where are your eyes?', 'Show me your finger', 'Where are your shoes?'. Alternatively a doll may be used as described in the Doll Vocabulary List (Sheridan, 1976) with instructions to 'Show me her hair' etc. In either case the requests should be given at a normal conversational level of voice initially and when satisfactory responses are obtained the voice should be lowered to 40 dB(A) and visual clues removed.

A combination of this and the previous techniques might help to secure the essential information about the child's ability to identify simple instructions at the minimal 40 dB(A) listening level and this then satisfies the first part of the test.

Some children who are developmentally slow, unco-operative, or who fail to respond in the first part of the test for other reasons, may need to be tested with the full distraction procedure outlined for the younger child. In such cases the facts should be noted in the child's records and the tester should question the parents very carefully about the child's expressive and receptive language usage at home. Included in the questioning should be:

'Can he/she understand simple instructions?' (request examples).
'Is he/she starting to put two or more words together?' (request examples).

AUDITORY ACUITY

In the second part of the test the distraction test is used to check that the child hears high frequency sounds at less than 35 dB(A). If possible the child's responses to middle and low frequencies should also be checked but for the mature child at this age it may be difficult to obtain more than two or three reliable responses with the distraction method. The problem here is that the mature child quickly weighs up the test situation and may turn once to satisfy his/her curiosity but thereafter inhibit further head turn responses.

The following tips may help to increase the number of responses.

Matching the sounds

By using the same stimulus sound at the front as part of the attention capture technique and then concealing it, this might motivate the child to turn out of curiosity when he/she hears it appear from behind.

Varying the order of presentation

To heighten novelty the sounds should be presented in varying order, for example, in the sequence 4 kHz warble, rattle, 's'. It may not be possible to obtain more than one response to each stimulus.

Figure 5.5: Duplicating stimuli in the distraction test

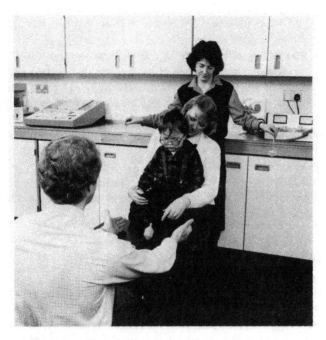

Prompting the response

If no response is forthcoming the distractor should say 'Where is the noise?' or 'Find the noise'. This will often provide the necessary motivation for the child to turn. It must be remembered, however, that 'no-sound' control trials should also be included with the same verbal prompting in order to observe the effects of this technique on normal searching behaviour.

Duplicated stimulus

The alert child who has weighed up the distraction situation will be more confused about the situation if warblers and rattles are held at both sides simultaneously as shown in Figure 5.5. Clearly the child cannot predict which stimulus will occur and with the inclusion of 'no-sound' control trials this arrangement should provide an excellent compromise.

PASS CRITERIA

If a child responds to the first part of the test, that is to the auditory discrimination part, at the minimal listening level and also to the high frequencies at less than 35 dB(A) in the second (distraction) part then this constitutes a pass. Checking the distraction responses for the middle and low frequencies clearly provides a more stringent test but this may not prove to be feasible for the reasons described. If, however, a child consistently fails to respond to the low or middle frequencies and yet can be shown to respond quickly and repeatedly to the high frequencies it would be worthwhile to retest the child again ensuring that a minimal level of voice is being used. The child should then be referred for diagnostic testing if the same pattern emerges and/or if there are any concerns about the speech and language development.

SUMMARY

The normal negative behaviour of the child between the ages of 18 months and 2½ years imposes unavoidable difficulties for the hearing screener. Nevertheless, with the range of tests described in this chapter, it is normally possible to extend the screening technique to include a measure of auditory discrimination in addition to auditory detection and this enables the screen to sample an aspect of everyday usage of hearing.

6

Testing the Hearing of Children with Mental Ages between Two-and-a-Half and Three-and-a-Half Years

By the time a child has developed a mental age of 2½ years he/she can usually exert a useful degree of voluntary control over certain impulses. The negative behaviour carried over from the latter half of the second year may persist through the first half of the third year but as the child approaches the age of 3 there may be more signs of a general willingness to please.

Simple operant conditioning techniques may be utilised within the test and these will be described under the section dealing with the performance test. As with the younger child's tests there are two parts to the hearing test for this age group: (a) screening auditory discrimination; and (b) screening auditory detection (acuity).

SCREENING AUDITORY DISCRIMINATION

Before describing the recommended procedure in full detail a general review of the 'speech discrimination' tests currently available in the UK will be given.

Stycar hearing tests (Sheridan, 1976)

The Stycar hearing tests devised by Dr Mary D. Sheridan consist of a series of graded toy and picture pointing tasks designed: 'to provide information regarding the presence of everyday auditory competence. They are basically clinical procedures evoking highly individualistic response and therefore not susceptible to sophisticated statistical evaluation.' Sheridan (1976).

Although the difficulties of standardising such tests for very young children are appreciated it is quite remarkable that despite very detailed accounts of the form of administration of the tests in the 60 page manual there is no mention of pass/fail criteria for the tests. In fact Dr Sheridan states: 'The terms 'pass' and 'fail' are not employed. The child is judged to respond or not respond according to the behavioural level of performance reasonably to be expected at his age.'

Despite the apparent sophistication of the selection of the toy and picture stimuli according to developmental guidelines there must be a serious shortcoming for any hearing screening test if a sound presentation level is not specified. The nearest approach to a guideline in the manual is that a 'quiet conversational' level should be used but this is not specified further and it is clearly a variable factor for different speakers. It is curious that although there is a lack of essential guidelines for a screening criterion in terms of the presentation level there is a very strict sequence for presentation of the material. For example, there are three toy tests (seven-toy, six-toy, and five-toy) and for each form the words must be delivered in a set order (e.g. spoon, doll, fork, car, knife, plane, and ship for the seven-toy).

The battery of tests also includes a doll vocabulary test and picture vocabulary tests in addition to word lists and sentence lists. With such a large array it is not surprising to find that people tend to choose an individual, preferred section for clinical application rather than work through the sequence of tests in the way advocated by Dr Sheridan.

RNID picture screening test for hearing (Reed, 1969)

This widely used test (shown in Figure 6.1) consists of eight flip-over test cards in a booklet, each with four pictures showing objects chosen to conform with the following conditions:

1. The words are monosyllabic so that the rhythm of the word does not give a clue.
2. The words on any card all contain the same vowel.
3. The words are within the vocabulary of children with a mental age of 4 years (e.g. the first card shows mouse, owl, cow and house).

The philosophy behind the choice of the items on individual cards is that if there is a slight loss of hearing for all frequencies

Figure 6.1: RNID picture screening test

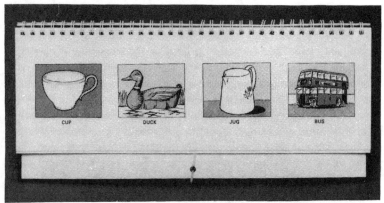

throughout the speech range, or severe loss for frequencies above 1 kHz there will be some disability in discriminating between consonants.

The instructions provided with the test specify no particular loudness level for presentation other than a 'conversational level' to condition the child, followed by a 'whispered voice' at 6 feet to test the child. The problem here is that a whisper can be anything from 30 dB or less up to 60 dB or more depending upon the individual and their interpretation of the task. Also, as already stated, the whisper distorts the acoustic relationships between sounds by removing the voicing characteristic.

The test could be improved by specifying a presentation level (for example 40 dB(A) as for the Kendall and McCormick tests) but to be fair to the original concept of the test it was designed for simple application by teachers and doctors who would not have access to sound-level meters etc. at a time when other tests were not available. The author, Michael Reed, claims that despite the fact that the test was designed for children with a mental age of 4 years and above it can also be used with many children of the mental age of 3 years. Undoubtedly this may be appropriate in some cases but few children of mental age 2½ years can cope with the vocabulary used in the test.

This test has been widely used but mostly for children above the age of 4 years and as such it is not ideally suited to cover the full age range of interest here which is from 2½ years upwards.

The Kendall toy test (Kendall, 1953, 1954)

The Kendall toy test in its original form consisted of three lists of 15 nouns (ten stimulus and five distractors) chosen to contain the common vowels and dipthongs in English and frequently occurring consonants. Each word has a toy representation and the test is administered by displaying one set of toys and requesting the child to point to the item spoken by the examiner.

Kendall originally developed three sets of toys intending that each should be presented at a different sound pressure level thus enabling a basic form of speech audiogram to be plotted showing the percentage score at differing listening levels. In fact, very few testers use the full form of the test and it is common to find just one of the lists being used and more often than not this is the third list containing the following:

test (stimulus) items: house, spoon, fish, duck, cow, shoe, brick, cup, gate, plate.

with the distraction items: mouse, book, string, glove, plane.

When the test is used in this way (which differs from Kendall's original design) there is no officially agreed pass/fail criterion although a tradition passed down over the years from the Department of Audiology, Manchester University, has been to present the words at 40 dB(A) and expect a consistently good score at that level for a screening pass.

The Dodds insert board (Dodds, 1972)

This test consists of a form board with a series of removable shapes depicting familiar everyday objects known to the average 3-year-old child. Only a very limited quantity of the tests has been produced and the advantages or limitations of the test remain to be assessed.

THE TOY DISCRIMINATION TEST (McCormick, 1977)

From the previous discussion it will be appreciated that no single test has proved to be entirely satisfactory for this age group. The Kendall toy test used in the modified form detailed above had for many years been the most widely used pre-school speech screening test in the UK but a more recent test developed by McCormick (1977) known as the 'toy discrimination test' has gradually gained in popularity having been developed for use with children with a mental age of 2 years and above. The similarity between the two tests is not surprising because the toy discrimination test was developed around the popular idea of using a single list of words whilst attempting to optimise the choice of words (1) in terms of their familiarity (for the child from a mental age of 2 years upwards), and (2) so that a maximum possible degree of acoustic similarity could exist between pairs of monosyllabic words in the list within the constraints imposed (a) by the very young child's limited vocabulary and (b) by the difficulty of obtaining suitable toy representations of the words in the list.

The toy discrimination test was developed in a clinical context over a 2-year period during which time those items from various vocabulary scales of young children which could be represented by simple toys were tested on children first, for ambiguity (for example dish, to match with fish, proved to be a poor item because it was variously known as bowl or saucer etc.) and secondly, for acoustic similarity with a paired item such that children with slight hearing disorders frequently confused the words. The final version of the test consists of the following seven pairs of toys:

cup	duck
spoon	shoe
man	lamb
plate	plane
horse	fork
key	tree
house	cow

The test is administered by setting out in a multiple display those paired items known to the child and requesting pointing responses as the names are spoken in a varying and unpredictable order. The pass/fail criterion is set at 40 dB(A) for *consistent* identification of the items that is, four correct responses out of five requests or 80 per cent. The full display is shown in Figure 6.2. Toy items were chosen, rather than pictures, for this test, because of their high interest factor and because the recognition of toys comes before the recognition of pictures in the developmental hierarchy. In addition, a selection of toys offers extreme versatility for the display enabling the number of toys and the organisation of the display to be varied

Figure 6.2: The toy discrimination test

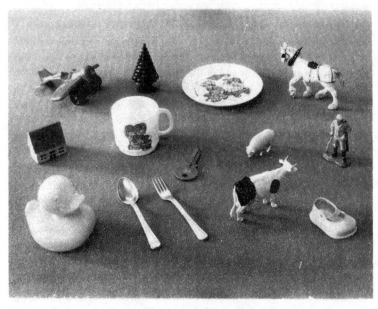

to suit the child's level of maturity, degree of co-operation, and perceptual span. From the list of toys it can be seen that each word has a matching item with a similar vowel or diphthong but differing consonants. Some children may wish to use the word sheep rather than lamb, gee rather than horse, and moo rather than cow, in which case there is a close similarity between the vowels in sheep, tree, key, gee and moo, shoe, spoon. The possibility of these and other alternatives should be taken into account during the administration of the test and also confusion of words with the same consonants but different vowels should be noted, for example house and horse.

Administration of the toy discrimination test

The child should be seated in a low chair adjacent to his/her parent or, alternatively, on the parent's lap if shy or withdrawn. The tester can kneel or be seated on a chair facing the table on which the toy display is to be established in front of the child (Figure 6.3). Each toy item can be brought out individually and the child encouraged to name it. This will permit an assessment to be made of the child's

Figure 6.3: The toy discrimination test situation

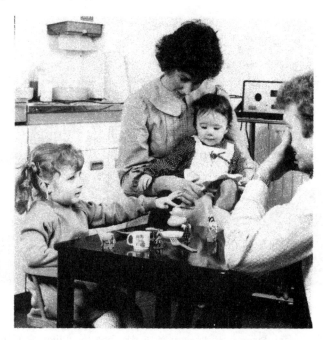

articulative skill and the tester should listen for the presence and quality of the high frequency consonants such as 's' and the consonant clusters such as 'tr' and 'pl'. Only those items clearly known to the child should be used. If the child is too shy or withdrawn to name the items at this stage of the test the parent should be asked to verify whether each item is known to the child and, if so, by what name. The number of items in the final display should be adjusted to suit the child's level of maturity but the final display should only contain matched pairs.

Having prepared a suitable display the tester can demonstrate to the child that he/she should point to each toy when he/she hears its name in the request 'Show me the . . .' or 'Where is the . . .?'. Alternatively the younger child might be asked to give the toy to mummy (or daddy) when asked to do so. Each toy must be returned to the display after each response. A conversational level of voice should be used at first until the child has a clear grasp of the task and then the tester should move to one side at one metre distance and the voice level should be lowered to the 40 dB(A) minimal level

Figure 6.4: Obtaining responses from the side

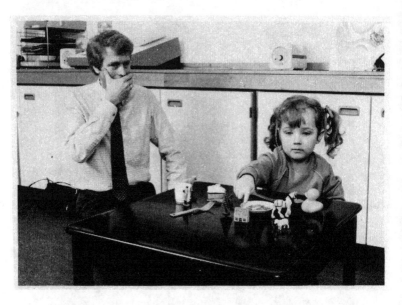

(without whispering) whilst covering the face to obliterate visual clues. Ideally responses should be obtained on each side at one metre distance from the ear and at right angles to the ear (Figure 6.4). In order to pass this screening test the child should respond correctly to four or more requests out of five presented at the 40 dB(A) minimal level on each side. Allowance may have to be made in the scoring if obvious drifts in the attention occur. Occasional repositioning of the toys on the table may help to recapture the attention sufficiently for a few additional responses to be obtained.

When testing shy children, withdrawn children, or children with motor difficulties, the toys can be spaced at reasonable distances apart so that eye pointing responses can be observed (see also the section on eye pointing in Chapter 5). When only a few items are used care should be taken to ensure that the instructions do not follow a set sequence. The choice of toy requested throughout the test should be haphazard and confusion patterns will be quite apparent if the child's hearing is not normal.

One of the great merits of a test of this kind is that the parent can observe directly the nature of the affected child's hearing problem. The child may be seen to respond well at the loud conversational level of voice but then be thoroughly confused when the voice level is lowered. Furthermore, the fact that the child may hear something at the quieter level, but may not discriminate correctly, can also be demonstrated and may help to provide the parent with a deeper understanding of the nature of the hearing problem. Some children will say 'what?' or 'pardon?' and may look in the direction of the speaker for visual clues and these are all useful pointers and typical behaviour characteristics of the child with hearing difficulties.

Criteria for passing the screening test

To pass the test the minimum acceptable response should be four correct identifications out of five instructions presented at 40 dB(A). It is strongly recommended that a sound-level meter be used to confirm that the minimal 40 dB(A) level is achieved. In the absence of a sound-level meter the guideline for attaining the level should be that an adult with normal hearing standing 3 metres away should be able to hear a faint speech signal but the clarity of the words should be indistinct.

If responses can be obtained from the front it cannot be assumed that both ears hear well. Ideally separate responses should be obtained on each side.

The advantages and limitations of the test

The chief advantage of this test is that it is very simple and can be used with children from a mental age of 2 years. Parents can observe the natural confusions which arise when a child has a slight hearing problem.

When correctly administered, the test can identify children who are quite definitely at risk because of hearing difficulty. The test does not, however, demonstrate absolute normality of hearing acuity and it is conceivable that some children with very slight high-tone or low-tone hearing loss might remain undetected, even though samples of their speech are heard. It is also conceivable that children with monaural hearing losses might pass the test. These children can sometimes be seen to strain to one side when listening on the poor side and the observant tester should be alert to these signs.

Despite the limitations of tests performed in a free field setting,

Figure 6.5: Items suitable for the performance test

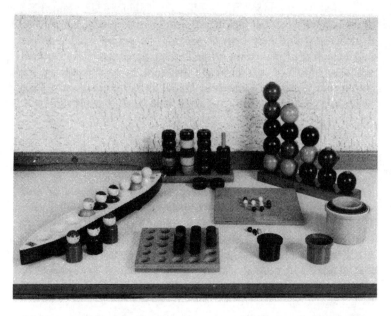

they are irreplaceable for the very young child and their value has been demonstrated clearly over many years.

SCREENING AUDITORS ACUITY — THE PERFORMANCE TEST

For this part of the test it is necessary to use simple play materials which offer the facility for the repetition of a simple task. A peg board, a ball on sticks, or men in a boat set as shown in Figure 6.5 would be ideal for this purpose.

The objective is to condition the child to respond by, for example, placing a man in the boat when a signal is presented and then utilise specific low and high frequency sounds to test the hearing in each ear. The traditional stimuli used in the past have been the word 'go' for low frequencies and the consonant 's' for high frequencies. These can be very effective if the presentation level is checked with a sound-level meter to ensure that the screening level of 35 dB or less is achieved. The 'go' will, however, contain a broad frequency band if the glottal stop 'g' is articulated and although it is acceptable to use the full word to establish the conditioning it will be necessary to reduce this to 'o' for the screen itself. Equally the 's' will only be valid as a high frequency sound if it is not forced or broadened to a 'sh' sound.

If warblers or narrow band noise makers are available these can be used to replace the 'go' and 's' stimuli and they clearly offer advantages in terms of standardisation and frequency specificity. With the younger child in this age group it may, however, be useful to use the 'go' stimulus to establish the initial conditioning and then to transfer to the electronic sounds later in the test.

Details of the conditioning procedure

One of the merits of this test is that it can be used without the need for verbal instruction. The conditioning can be established by demonstration only and this clearly has advantages for application with children from ethnic minorities who may have language difficulties. Having chosen a toy item suitable for the child's level of maturity the tester should first demonstrate the 'game' by:

1. holding a peg over the board (Figure 6.6);
2. waiting for the stimulus;
3. inserting the peg in the board when the stimulus is presented, and
4. rewarding the response with, for example, a hand clap.

A few demonstration responses of this nature should be presented with the stimulus sound of choice at a moderately high loudness level and with visual clues such as a head nod to reinforce the response. If warblers are used they should be held near to the ear to achieve the loud level at this stage of the test. It might be useful to let the child's parent participate in the game before finally inviting the child to hold one of the pegs. Gentle restraint and guidance of the child's hand may be needed at first (Figure 6.7):

1. to avoid premature responses;
2. to sense whether the child is responding correctly to the stimulus; and
3. to guide the response promptly when the stimulus is presented if no timely reaction is present from the child. It is very important to reward correct responses and hence provide the necessary

85

Figure 6.6: Demonstrating the performance test activity

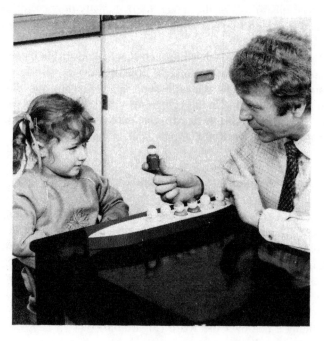

degree of positive reinforcement to retain the child's interest and co-operation.

If the child is developmentally ready for the task reliable conditioning should be established after the first five or so demonstrations. As a general rule, if no signs of restraint are apparent after 20 guided demonstrations it is unlikely that the test will be appropriate and it may be necessary to resort to distraction techniques.

Avoiding visual clues

Once the conditioning has been established at moderately loud levels, aided by visual cueing, the visual cues should be removed and the stimulus level should be lowered to 35 dB(A) or less. In practice this means that if a warbler is used it should be held at the maker's recommended distance set back from the ear at an angle of 45° (Figure 6.8). The child must not be permitted to watch the movement of the tester's hand (or arm) as the stimulus is presented.

Figure 6.7: Guiding the child's response

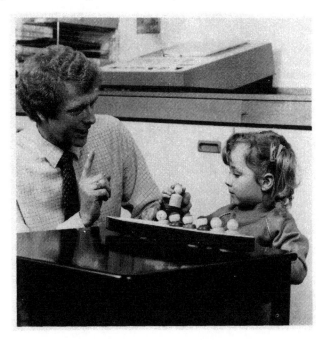

If the 'go' or 's' stimuli are used the child must not be permitted to look in the direction of the tester because there will always be some visual whole body, limb, head, mouth, or eyebrow clues present when the sounds are made. Covering the face is not recommended for this test and the rule is that the child should not be permitted to look in the direction of the tester. The tester should be at arm's length from the child, set back at an angle of 45° to avoid such cueing when using the 'go' and 's' sounds (Figure 6.9).

Varying the timing of stimulus presentation

It is important to avoid establishing a situation in which the child responds to the stimulus in a set rhythm. This can be avoided by varying the timing of the stimulus presentation in a haphazard fashion such that the child may have to wait anything from between 1 and 10 seconds before the sound appears. The long waits are the ones which provide a useful check on the child's state of attention.

Figure 6.8: Using a warbler for the performance test

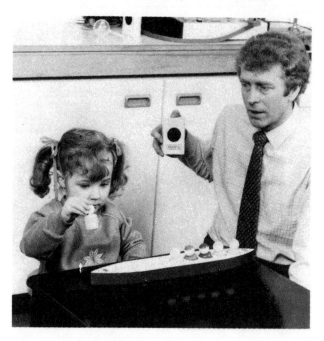

Reconditioning for stimulus change

It cannot be assumed that a child will readily transfer the conditioning from one stimulus to another and, particularly with the younger child, it is wise to present a few guided responses when introducing each new stimulus.

When transferring from the 'go' to the 's' stimulus it is not unusual for a child to articulate 'go' before responding to each 's' stimulus and this is not surprising given the nature of the 'go' command.

Criteria for passing the test

To pass the test the child should respond to three low frequency ('go', 500 Hz warble or narrow band) stimuli and three high frequency ('s', or 4 kHz warble tone, or narrow band) stimuli in each ear at the minimal level of less than 35 dB. If warblers are used it will be useful to add a mid-frequency stimulus. Responses should occur for each trial at the minimal level unless there are obvious drifts in the child's attention. Attention lapses and ambient noise

Figure 6.9: Position for presenting the 'go' and 's' stimuli

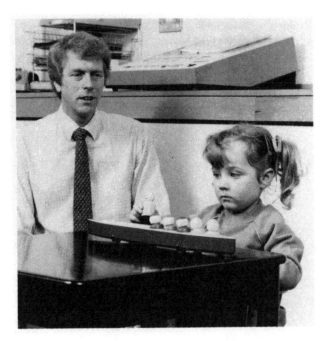

disturbances in the test environment are often unavoidable and they not only prolong the timing of the test but also pose problems in the formulation of the test structure in terms of the number of specified trials. All that can be stated is that the tester should introduce sufficient trials to be certain that at least four consistent responses occur out of five presentations at the minimal level. The variable delay in the presentation of the stimulus provides a useful measure of the consistency particularly during the long delay intervals.

Simple forms can be used to record the results of the test showing 'pass' or 'refer for further testing' for the right and left ears for each of the stimuli available.

The choice of screening level must be made according to local policy. In Nottingham we recommend the use of 25 dB or 30 dB(A) if warblers are used, depending upon the setting available on the model used. For the conventional 'go' and 's' sounds it is unrealistic to expect that a screening level of less than 35 dB(A) will be achieved in practice.

SUMMARY

The increased sophistication in the child's development in the third year of life is reflected in the hearing screening test technique which now makes use of simple conditioning and an extended range of toy materials.

7

The Sound-Level Meter and Room Acoustics

THE INSTRUMENTS

Whenever hearing tests are performed it is highly desirable to have some means of measuring the environmental noise and the level of the stimuli used in the test. For screening purposes very basic low cost instruments are acceptable and it is not necessary to invest in costly meters containing a wide range of facilities. The simple instrument, shown in Figure 7.1, has a microphone mounted at one end and a moving needle meter which can be adjusted to record sound levels ranging from 35 dB(A) to 130 dB(A) according to the position of the sensitivity switch. If, for example, the switch is set at 40 dB the meter will read from 40 dB − 5 dB (35 dB) up to 40 dB + 10 dB (50 dB).

This instrument also has a slow and fast response option. In the slow response position the needle response is more 'damped' and does not fluctuate rapidly with varying sounds. This setting is used for monitoring an averaged level of a fluctuating long-term sound such as running speech. When recording sound levels in the hearing screening tests described in this book it will be more appropriate to use the 'fast' response setting for the short duration sounds of interest.

The remaining switch on the instrument shown in Figure 7.1 is for turning it on and off and for checking the battery. If the battery has the correct voltage the needle should deflect to the 'battery test' area on the dial, otherwise a replacement battery will be needed.

An alternative instrument which utilises a light-emitting diode flying dot display is shown in Figure 7.2. The use of silicon chip technology has helped to increase the robustness of the instrument and also reduce cost. The instrument in Figure 7.2 shares the

Figure 7.1: Simple sound-level meter

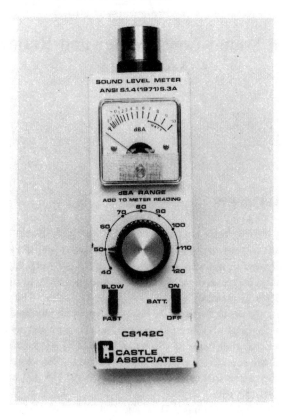

features of that in Figure 7.1 but the display is calibrated in 3 dB steps rather than 1 dB on the moving needle meter. These 3 dB steps are perfectly adequate for hearing screening purposes.

MEASURING SOUNDS

The microphone of the sound-level meter represents the child's ear and strictly speaking should be mounted in the position occupied by the child's ear during the test. This is clearly not possible because the child's head would have to be moved to make way for the sound level meter. A compromise situation is called for when using such instruments in a clinical context and the recommendation is that the microphone of the meter should be positioned at the same distance

Figure 7.2: Sound-level indicator

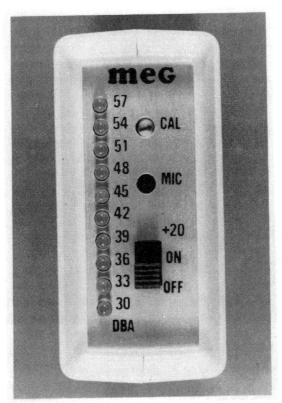

from the sound as the child's ear. Ideally the meter should be mounted adjacent to the child's head as shown in Figure 7.3 and each sound should be checked for level. The background noise should also be measured at the position occupied by the child's head during the test. Slight inaccuracies can be expected when using meters in the way described here because the presence of the child in the sound field influences that sound field to a certain degree. The errors are, however, of such acceptably small magnitude as to be negligible in the hearing screening context.

If pre-calibrated warblers or other electronic noise makers are used it should not be necessary to measure the levels with a sound-level meter during a test but the devices must, of course, be used at the correct distance. As a general rule, for the distances used in the tests described in this book, each halving of distance will increase

Figure 7.3: Position for holding the sound-level meter

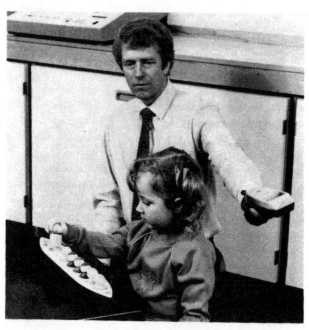

the sound pressure level by 6 dB and therefore errors of a few centimetres at the normal 50 cm distance for warblers will be in the order of a decibel or so. The same consideration applies to errors in distance placement of sound-level meters.

However desirable it might be to measure each sound with a meter during the test this ideal is rarely achieved in reality and the meter is often just used to calibrate the tester from time to time. This problem usually arises because of the lack of availability of sufficient instruments to provide one for each tester. The need for regular calibration of testers and annual calibration checks for sound-level meters and warblers cannot be over-emphasised.

REQUIREMENTS FOR THE TEST ROOM

The ideal room for undertaking the tests described in this book would satisfy the following requirements:

1. Minimum dimension 4 m × 4 m.
2. Furnishings to include carpet and curtains or blinds.
3. Quiet situation free from intermittent or constant external noise from car parks, corridors, waiting rooms, staff rooms, etc.
4. Calm uncluttered atmosphere without too many visual distractions.
5. Background noise level not exceeding 35 dB(A).

Most of these requirements are fairly obvious apart from the background noise level which needs further discussion.

Acoustic requirements of the test room

Background (or ambient) noise in a test room should not exceed certain values to avoid masking the test sounds. Problems arise in specifying the permissable noise level first, because the noise may fluctuate and secondly, because the masking effect depends upon certain characteristic acoustic features of the noise.

Intermittent vs. constant noise

A constant noise of 50 dB in a test room would be unacceptable but the same may not apply if the noise is intermittent in nature. Intermittent noise levels of 50 dB will be measurable in most test rooms and the factor which will determine whether the room is suitable for testing will be the frequency of occurrence of such sounds. If the sounds only appear every minute or so there will be sufficient quiet periods for the testing to take place. More frequent bursts of noise would not be acceptable but the odd burst of noise every minute or so would simply prolong the test because any responses recorded from the child which coincided with the noise would have to be disregarded.

When assessing the suitability of a room for hearing test purposes the ambient noise level should be measured during a typical quiet interval if such intervals have an average duration of more than a minute.

The acoustic characteristic of ambient noise

It is possible that a room with an ambient noise level in excess of 35 dB(A) is suitable for hearing test purposes using stimuli of 35 dB(A). This may appear to be an impossible situation but the explanation is simply that the acoustic characteristic of the masking

95

Figure 7.4: Mean background noise levels in community clinics (*n* = 27), the dotted lines either side of the mean show plus and minus one standard deviation

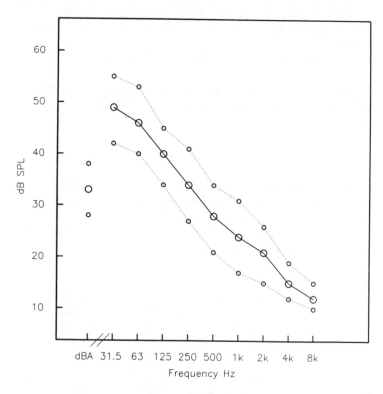

noise is the dependent factor. To be certain about the effects of a particular noise it is necessary to undertake an octave band analysis to determine its frequency distribution. An analysis of this nature undertaken by the writer in 27 community hearing test locations in Nottinghamshire is shown in Figure 7.4. The sound pressure level at octave intervals across the frequency range from 31.5 Hz to 8 kHz is shown. The equipment required to undertake this analysis is rather costly and would not normally be available in a community health service. The measurements are obtained in octave intervals by filtering out sounds not contained within the octave of interest. It can be seen that most of the ambient noise in these community test locations occurs at low frequencies below 500 Hz and despite the fact that some very low-frequency sounds are reaching 50 dB the mean sound level for the 27 rooms is only 32.7 dB. For the frequencies of interest for hearing screening purposes, that is between 500 Hz and 4 kHz, the components of the noise are well below 30 dB.

In the absence of the appropriate octave band filtering equipment it is possible to check the suitability of a room by performing a simple psycho-acoustical test. This is performed by taking two or more people with known normal hearing and checking that the stimuli can be heard at the appropriate distance. Although this may appear to be a rather crude check it does work very well in practice.

SUMMARY

Hearing tests will not achieve a respectable degree of validity and reliability unless the intensity of the stimuli used and the background noise levels are measured. The simple inexpensive instruments available for this purpose have been described in this chapter. The general recommendation is that the level of the stimuli and the ambient noise should not exceed 35 dB(A). In many situations it may, however, be possible to apply the test in ambient noise levels in excess of 35 dB(A) if it can be confirmed that the most intense components of the noise occur at frequencies well below 500 Hz as is normally the case.

8

The Future — New Methods on the Horizon

A PERSPECTIVE

This book has concentrated on behavioural hearing screening methods which do not require highly sophisticated and expensive equipment. Methods are currently being evaluated which are considered to be more objective in the sense that human observation is replaced by, for example, electrical recording of physiological or behavioural responses to sound. Such methods are already used in diagnostic clinical and laboratory settings but it is only in recent years that attention has turned to the utilisation of the methods in a screening context. Clearly it takes years rather than months to evaluate such methods on large numbers of babies and to collect the necessary follow-up data to compile sensitivity and specificity ratings for each method.

It is unlikely that the advent of the newer more objective methods will completely replace the need for the behavioural methods discussed in this book. What is more likely is that they will complement the current methods and perhaps enable congenital deafness to be detected at the neonatal stage. There will still be a need for a hearing screening test to be performed during the first year of life to detect not only the false negative cases from neonatal testing but also cases of progressive deafness and cases of acquired sensori-neural or conductive deafness.

The progress and change in the objective test field is so rapid that the content of this chapter will become out of date much more rapidly than the coverage of the behavioural methods included earlier. Nevertheless an illustration of the type of research which is underway will be given. This coverage is designed to be illustrative rather than exhaustive.

THE AUDITORY RESPONSE CRADLE (ARC)

It is known that newborn babies react to sound by showing responses such as, for example, startles, head turns and changes in respiration. These responses could not be interpreted reliably prior to the advent of microprocessor technology because of the high degree of spontaneous activity in the awake baby and because of observer bias. The ARC was developed by Dr M.J. Bennett as a microprocessor-controlled device to detect hearing responses against a background of spontaneous activity (Bennett, 1975). The device consists of a trolley, of similar size to a normal neonatal cradle, which houses a microprocessor and associated electronics beneath a moulded plastic cradle. The microprocessor records and saves information from a series of non-invasive pressure activated transducers which monitor the baby's head turns, head jerks (startles), body activities and respiration movements at times when sound stimuli are presented and also during blank trial periods when no sound stimuli are presented. The ARC passes or fails a baby by checking the recorded responses against a decision table which compares the number of responses during sound trials with those in the control trials. The sound trials used are broad band high pass noise (2.6–4.4 kHz) of high intensity (85 dB SPL), this being the level required to elicit behavioural changes in question.

The ARC is being evaluated in various centres in the United Kingdom and elsewhere. Following earlier work by McCormick, Curnock and Spavins (1984) and Davis (1984) various modifications and improvements have been made to the unit used at Nottingham and the Nottingham team is continuing to develop better and more reliable recording devices. It will take several years to complete multi-centre trials and only tentative conclusions can be drawn about the ARC and other devices of its kind. The technique has the great merit of being non-invasive and, furthermore, it has the virtue of recording the total behavioural response to sound rather than just sampling a very limited physiological response.

BRAINSTEM AUDITORY EVOKED RESPONSE MEASUREMENTS (BSER)

Brainstem Auditory Evoked Response (BSER) recordings utilising auditory stimuli have been used for many years in diagnostic audiology clinics and they are accepted as part of the routine battery

99

of tests available to audiologists. Historically the instrumentation used has been very expensive requiring a high level of technical skill to use, and the test has been time-consuming often needing sedation and other special facilities. More recently, simplified forms of the test have been devised for use in a screening context with particular emphasis on neonates.

Brainstem evoked response audiometry (sometimes termed electric response audiometry or ERA) is an objective non-invasive method of evaluating auditory function and as such it has application for use with the very young. Essentially the method consists of recording changes in the brain's EEG activity in response to sound. The auditory brainstem response comprises up to seven vertex-positive electrical waves generated in the cochlear nerve and subsequent neurones of the auditory pathway up to the mid-brain, usually occurring within 10 ms of stimulus onset. The evoked responses can be detected by means of electrodes mounted on the surface of the scalp and auditory threshold measurements are usually based on the computer averaged wave-five response since it can be detected within 10 dB of the behavioural threshold for mature subjects or in the region of 30 dB or 40 dB in the case of the neonate.

With anticipated further technical improvements and refinements in waveform analysis it can be assumed that BSER methods will be utilised widely in neonatal screening programmes in years to come. It must, however, be borne in mind that the method does not test the entire hearing pathway to the same degree as the behavioural methods and caution must be exercised in interpreting such electrophysiological data. The stimuli used for the test normally consist of clicks which are centred in the frequency region between 2.5 kHz and 3 kHz. Further refinements will be needed before the test can sample responses in the low speech frequency region.

RECORDING THE POST-AURICULAR MYOGENIC (PAM) RESPONSE

The PAM response was first described by Kiang, Crist, French and Edwards (1963). The principle is that when sounds are presented to the ears a minute response can be recorded in the post-auricular muscle. In certain animals, for example dogs, the response can be observed as ear pricking behaviour but in man the overt outward signs are invisible and electrophysiological means are needed to record the electrical potential generated in the muscle using the now-familiar computer averaging principle (see section on BSER). The PAM response has a large amplitude and a long latency period (15 ms) relative to other evoked responses and these characteristics make it fairly easy to detect. Also general muscular movement enhances the appearance of response rather than tending to extinguish it and this makes it suitable for application to young or unco-operative subjects without the need for sedation.

Various studies have been made to assess the usefulness of the PAM response for hearing assessment purposes (Douek, Gibson and Humphries, 1973; Thornton, 1975) and more recently the technique has been used with infants (Fraser, Conway, Keene and Hazell, 1978; Flood, Fraser, Conway and Stewart, 1982). The technique consists of recording an electrical evoked response to sound from surface electrodes positioned in the pre- and post-auricular skin areas of one ear using a third electrode, often positioned at the back of the neck, as an earth. Click stimuli are presented to the ear either from a speaker or earphone and the resulting electrical potentials recorded from the post-auricular muscle and averaged over several hundred or several thousand click stimuli.

The PAM response has bilateral representation, that is stimulation of one ear will elicit the response in both post-auricular muscles, and it is sometimes referred to as the Crossed Acoustic Response.

Flood et al. (1982) designed a portable screening device for recording the PAM response known as the Body Spek 2000. This equipment has been evaluated in numerous screening programmes, including one organised by the writer at Nottingham. In its original form the equipment presents click stimuli with a choice of two loudness levels of 60 dB (HL) and 80 dB (HL). It has, however, been found that a number of babies with conductive hearing losses and adults with sensori-neural hearing losses in the region of 30/40 dB actually pass the test at the 60 dB (HL) PAM level. This is not unexpected in view of the fact that the PAM response can be recorded down to 0 dB (HL). The writer did not consider this to be satisfactory for screening purposes and with the co-operation of the manufacturer a revised form of the equipment with 40, 50 and 60 dB (HL) click stimuli is being evaluated. The results of these early trials have indicated that the designer's claims for the unit are substantiated when they stated 'We feel that the PAM screening test should not be considered in isolation, but as a useful adjunct to existing tests where there is still doubt about the hearing.'

There are two main reasons why the PAM test may not be robust or reliable enough for application as an independent screening method:

1. There is a considerable degree of inter- and intra-subject variability in the appearance of the PAM response.
2. The equipment in its present form does not sample responses at different frequencies. Clicks are essentially high pass noise stimuli. However, subjects with very significant high frequency hearing loss can still remain undetected if a high stimulus presentation level of 60 dB (HL) or 80 dB (HL) is used.

MIDDLE EAR IMPEDANCE MEASUREMENTS

Middle ear impedance readings are incorporated routinely in diagnostic audiology clinics and they serve a valuable function by, on the one hand, determining the normality of the middle ear mechanical and pneumatic function and, on the other hand, recording the integrity of the nerve pathways up to brainstem level utilising the contraction of the stapedius muscle. The technique involves inserting an earprobe in the external auditory canal. This probe is connected to a transmitter, which sends a soundwave along the ear canal, and a receiver which records the reflection of this soundwave from the eardrum (tympanic membrane). The air pressure in the canal and therefore the pressure loading on the eardrum is varied by means of a pump and the pressure is measured using a manometer arrangement. The mobility of the eardrum and the pressure within the middle ear space can be deduced by recording the changes in the reflectivity of the sound as the pressure in the canal is varied. Clearly a positive or negative pressure loading will tense the drum and produce a high reflectivity and a balanced pressure loading, such that the pressures in the canal and middle ear space are equal, will result in a low reflectivity reading because the drum will lack tension and the sound will be absorbed. Any changes in the vibration characteristics of the ossicular chain brought about, for example, by the contraction of the stapedial muscle which pulls on the stapes, will influence the degree to which sound is absorbed or reflected by the drum, hence the use of the technique for recording the contraction of the stapedial reflex.

There has been considerable debate about the general appropriateness of the technique in a screening context. Very few workers would recommend the use of the technique in isolation from other methods. One of the main reservations relates to the extreme sensitivity of the recordings and the susceptibility of the middle ear to show minor transient changes in the absence of medically significant pathology or educationally significant hearing threshold variation.

Until more normative studies have been completed it will not be possible to establish clear pass/fail criteria from middle ear impedance measurements which fit well within the context of hearing screening for babies. The technique measures pathology rather than hearing and it is recommended that such measurements should retain their rightful place in diagnostic clinics rather than in hearing screening programmes.

RECORDING OTOACOUSTIC EMISSIONS

The recording of weak echoes from the cochlea in response to sounds presented to the ear was first reported by Kemp (1978). The echo is called an otoacoustic emission and it is believed to arise from the active biomechanics of the cochlear sensory mechanism at a pre-neural level. It can be recorded in response to a pulsed stimulus by means of a sealed probe microphone positioned in the ear canal. Kemp demonstrated, with the aid of computer averaging techniques and acoustic stimuli lasting tens of milliseconds, that the emissions were present in ears with normal hearing but they were absent in ears with sensori-neural hearing losses in excess of 30 dB (HL). The response pattern differs significantly from one ear to another both with regard to the number of echoes and their appearance items (latencies) and their intensity and frequency content, but they are reported to produce stable patterns for each individual.

Three classes of emissions can be identified:

1. *Spontaneous emissions.* These are usually tones which come from many normal ears and are sometimes heard by the subject as mild tinnitus.
2. *Stimulus frequency emissions.* These are echoes of the stimulus presented to the ear arising from within the cochlea. They are present whenever the stimulus is present.
3. *Intermodulation or product emissions.* These are present whenever complex sounds (e.g. simultaneous presentation of two similar frequencies) are used.

The echoes are very weak, hence the need for computer-assisted averaging of several hundred or several thousand responses using identical signal averaging principles to those used in Brain Stem Evoked Response Recordings. The echoes usually produce a peak

103

response some 8–12 ms after stimulation and for stimulus frequency emissions it lasts 15 ms whereas in the case of spontaneous emissions the echo may last 50 ms.

The tests in perspective

It will be appreciated from this introduction to the technique that this objective test requires very complex instrumentation and sensitive recording apparatus. Johnsen, Bagi and Elberling (1983) demonstrated that the technique could be applied to neonates with a test time per case of approximately 10 minutes. There are, however, several problems still to be overcome, not the least of which is the prerequisite that the technique can only be applied in cases where completely normal middle ear function exists. More research is needed to define normative data for neonates and infants middle ear function and the effect of this on otoacoustic emission recordings. The degree to which the technique can provide information about the ear's response to different frequencies is uncertain and needs further investigation.

The results of field trials are awaited with great interest and if the outcome from these are favourable this test could be a serious contender for screening neonates or difficult to test children. The particular merits of the test are the short test time and the non-invasive nature of the test.

SUMMARY

Examples of the newer more objective tests have been presented and the fact that these are still at the evaluation stage has been stressed. A common limitation of any test which does not record a full behavioural response to sound is that only a certain part of the auditory pathway is being assessed. Although it may be stated that a sound has arrived at that particular site, it cannot be assumed that there has been a processing beyond that site. Given that objective tests share this limitation it may be that a combination of methods utilising the strengths of behavioural and physiological responses will provide the best option for the future.

References

Bender, R. (1967) A child's hearing: Part II. Evaluation of a child's hearing. *Maico Audiological Library Series*, *3*, 4–7

Bennett, M.J. (1975) The auditory response cradle: a device for the objective assessment of auditory state in the neonate. *Symposia of the Zoological Society of London*, *37*, 291–305

Boothman, R. and Orr, N. (1978) Value of screening for deafness in first year of life. *Archives of Disease in Childhood*, *53*, 570–3

Dalzell, J. and Owrid, H.L. (1976) Children with conductive deafness — a follow up study. *British Journal of Audiology*, *10*, 87–90

Davis, A. (1984) The statistical decision criterion for the auditory response cradle. *British Journal of Audiology*, *18*, 163–8

DHSS (1981) Department of Health and Social Security Advisory Committee on Services for Hearing-Impaired People. Final report of the sub-committee appointed to consider services for hearing impaired children. June 1981

Dodds, J. (1972) An object puzzle as an indicator of hearing acuity. *Sound*, *6*, 49–55

Douek, E., Gibson, W. and Humphries, K. (1973) The crossed acoustic response. *Journal of Laryngology and Otology*, *87*, 711–26

Downs, M. (1981) Contributions of mild hearing loss to auditory learning problems. In R. Roeser and M. Downs (eds), *Disorders in school children*, Theime-Stratton, New York, pp. 176–89

Eisenberg, R.B. (1965) Examination of auditory behaviour. *Journal of Auditory Research*, *5*, 159–77

Ewing, I.R. and Ewing, A.W.G. (1944) The ascertainment of deafness in infancy and early childhood. *Journal of Laryngology and Otology*, *59*, 309–38

Ewing, I.R. and Ewing, A.W.G. (1947) *Opportunity and the deaf child*, University of London Press

Flood, L.M., Fraser, J.G., Conway, M.J. and Stewart, A. (1982) The assessment of hearing in infancy using the post-auricular myogenic response. *British Journal of Audiology*, *16*, 211–14

Fraser, G.R. (1976) *The cause of profound deafness in childhood*, The Johns Hopkins University Press, Baltimore

Fraser, J.G., Conway, M.J., Keene, M.H. and Hazell, J.W.P. (1978) The post-auricular myogenic response. *Journal of Laryngology and Otology*, *92*, 293–303

Froescels, E. and Beebe, H. (1946) Testing the hearing of newborn infants. *Archives of Otolaryngology*, *44*, 710–14

Gerber, S.E. and Mencher, G.T. (1978) *Early diagnosis of hearing loss*, Grune and Stratton, New York

Haggard, M.P. and Gannon, M.M. (1985) Analysis from service records of screening systems for hearing-impairment in pre-school children, *Medical Research Council Institute of Hearing Research Internal Report Series A, No. 3*, November 1985

Haggard, M.P. and Robinson, S. (1986) Middle ear disease and auditory disability in childhood' (in press)

Hamilton, P. (1972) Language and reading skills in children with impaired hearing in ordinary schools. Unpublished M.Ed. Thesis, University of Manchester

Health Visitor's Association (1977) *A survey of hearing testing undertaken by health visitors.* Health Visitors' Association, London

Hitchings, V. and Haggard, M.P. (1983) Incorporation of parental suspicion in screening infants hearing. *British Journal of Audiology, 17,* 71–5

Howie, V.M., Ploussard, J.H. and Slayer, J. (1975) The 'otitis-prone' condition. *American Journal of Diseases in Childhood, 129,* 676–780

Jaffe, B.F. (1977) *Hearing loss in children,* University Park Press, Baltimore

Jerger, S., Jerger, J., Alford, B.R. and Abrams, S. (1983) Development of speech and intelligibility in children with recurrent otitis media. *Ear and Hearing, 4,* 138–45

Johnsen, N.J., Bagi, P. and Elberling, C. (1983) Evoked acoustic emission from the human ear. *Scandinavian Audiology, 12,* 17–24

Kemp, D.T. (1978) Stimulated acoustic emissions from within the human auditory system. *Journal Acoustical Society America, 64,* 1386–91

Kendall, D.C. (1953) Audiometry for young children. *Teacher of the Deaf, 306,* 171–7

Kendall, D.C. (1954) Audiometry for young children. *Teacher of the Deaf, 307,* 18–23

Kiang, N.Y.S., Crist, A.H., French, M.A. and Edwards, A.G. (1963) *Quarterly Progress Report,* Laboratory of Electronics, Massachusetts Institute of Technology, vol. 68, p. 218

Klein, J.O., Bess, F.M., Bluestone, C.D. and Harford, E.R. (1978) *Impedance screening for middle-ear disease in children,* New York, Grune and Stratton

Latham, A.D. and Haggard, M.P. (1980) A pilot study to detect hearing impairment in the young. *Midwife, Health Visitor, and Community Nurse, 16,* 370–4

Lilholdt, T., Courtois, J. and Kortholm, B. (1980) The diagnosis of negative middle ear pressures in children. *Acta otolaryngologica, 89,* 459–64

Ling, D., Ling, A. and Doehring, D. (1970) Stimulus responses and observer variables in the auditory screening of newborn infants. *Journal of Speech and Hearing Research, 13,* 9–18

McCormick, B. (1977) The toy discrimination test: an aid for screening the hearing of children above a mental age of two years. *Public Health, London, 91,* 67–73

McCormick, B. (1983) Hearing screening by health visitors: a critical appraisal of the distraction test. *Health Visitor, 56,* 449–51

McCormick, B. (1986) Evaluation of a warbler in hearing screening tests. *Health Visitor, 59,* 143-4

McCormick, B., Curnock, D.A. and Spavins, F. (1984) Auditory screening of special care neonates using the auditory response cradle. *Archives of Disease in Childhood, 59,* 1168–72

McCormick, B., Wood, S.A., Cope, Y. and Spavins, F.M. (1984) Analysis of records from an open access audiology service. *British Journal of Audiology*, *18*, 127–32

Martin, J.A.M., Bentzen, O., Colley, J.R.T., Hennebert, D., Holm, C., Iurato, S., de Jonge. G.A. McCullen, O., Meyer, M.L., Moore, W.J. and Morgan, A. (1981) Childhood deafness in the European Community. *Scandinavian Audiology*, *10*, 165

Martin, J.A.M. and Moore, W.J. (1979) Childhood deafness in the European Community, *EUR 5413*, Commission of the European Communities, Luxembourg

Mendel, M.I. (1968) Infant responses to recorded sounds. *Journal of Speech and Hearing Research*, *11*, 811–16

Menyuk, P. (1977) Effects of hearing loss on language acquisition in the babbling stage. In B.F. Jaffee (ed.), *Hearing loss in children*, University Park Press, Baltimore, pp. 621–9

National Deaf Children's Society (1983) *Discovering deafness*, NDCS, London

Northern, J.L. and Downs, M.P. (1982) *Hearing in children*. William and Wilkins, Baltimore

Paradise, J. (1983) Long-term effects of short-term hearing loss — menace or myth? In *Effects of Otitis Media on the Child, Pediatrics*, *71*, 639–52

Pukander, J., Karma, P. and Sipila, M. (1982) Occurrence and recurrence of acute otitis media amongst children. *Acta Otolaryngologica*, *94*, 479–86

Rapin, I. (1978) Consequences of congenital hearing loss — A long term view. *Journal of Otolaryngology*, *7*, 473–83

Reed, M. (1969) *RNID Picture Screening Test of hearing*. Royal National Institute for the Deaf, 105 Gower Street, London

Sheridan, M.D. (1976) *Manual for the Stycar hearing tests*. National Federation for Educational Research Publishing Co. Ltd, 2 Jennings Buildings, Thames Avenue, Windsor

Simmons, F.B. (1978) Identification of hearing loss in infants and young children. *Otolaryngology Clinics of North America*, *11*, 19

Tervoort, B. (1964) Development of language and critical periods in the young deaf child: Identification and management. *Acta Otolaryngology (Stockholm)*, *206*, 247–55

Thornton, A.R.D. 91975) The use of post-auricular muscle response. *Journal of Laryngology and Otology*, *89*, 997–1010

Tucker, I. and Nolan, M. (1984) *Educational audiology*, Croom Helm, London

Index

acoustic neuromas 17
adenoidectomy 14
air-bone gap 11
Alport's syndrome 11
anoxia 19
antihistamines 14
Apert's syndrome 13, 18
apnoeic attacks 19
atresia 13, 17
audiogram 4–9
  audiometric threshold 4, 9
  configurations 5–9, 10–12
audiometry 9, 25–6
  air conduction 9–10
  bone conduction 9–10
  bone vibrator 10
  masking 11
auditory nerve 9
auditory response cradle 99

background (ambient) noise 26,
  88–9, 91–7
brain abscess 16
brainstem auditory evoked
  response 99–100
brittle bone disease (osteogenesis
  imperfecta) 18

cerebral palsy 16
cholesteatoma 16
cleft palate 13, 19
cochlea 9
cochlea echoes 103–4
cochlea implants 25
Cockayne syndrome 18
co-operative test 65, 68
Crouzon's syndrome 13, 18
cytomegalovirus 16, 19

decibel (dB) 4
decongestants 14
distraction test 23–4, 44–64
  age 46
  economics 45
  equipment 47

  maturation 58
  no sound trials 61
  organisation 47
  pass criteria 58–63
  personnel 47
  record forms 58–60
  record of success 44–5
  requirements 46–64
  response reinforcement 61
  space 47
  timing 52, 54, 62
Dodd's insert board 78
Down's syndrome 18–19

eardrum *see tympanic membrane*
encephalitis 16, 20
eustachian tube 13–14
external auditory meatus 9, 13

four-toy eyepointing test 66

genetic disorders 17–20
glue ear 14, 25
goitre 18
Goldenhar's syndrome 13
grommet 14

head trauma 17, 20
hearing loss 5, 9
  acquired 16
  causes 12–20
  conductive 9–11, 13–16
  congenital 16
  high tone 5, 27, 43, 83
  sensori-neural 9–12, 16–20
hearing screening 21–4, 26–7,
  33, 55, 65, 89
  definitions 21–4
  false negative 22
  false positive 22
  levels 26–7, 33, 55, 65, 89
  screening 23
  sensitivity 21–2
  specificity 21–2
  surveillance 24

testroom requirements 94–7
Hertz (definition) 1–2
high frequency rattle 31–2, 55–6
Hunter's syndrome 18
hyperbilirubinaemia 19

Kendall toy test 78
Klippel-Feil syndrome 13, 18

mastoid bone 10
maternal rubella 16, 19
measles 16
Ménière's disease 17
meningitis 16, 20
middle ear 9
    infections 13, 19
    malformations 13
    pressure 102
middle ear impedance
    measurements 102–3
mumps 16, 20
myringoplasty operation 13
myringotomy operation 14

octave band analysis 95
ossicles 9
    fixation 13
    ossicular chain 10
    staples 9, 13
otitis media 9, 19, 24–5
    acute suppurative 13–14, 25
    serous 14, 19
    secretory 13
otoacoustic emissions 103–4
otosclerosis 13, 16
ototoxic drugs 17, 19
    colistin 19
    gentamycin 19
    kanamycin 19
    streptomycin 19
oval window 9–10, 13

Paget's disease 13
Pendred's syndrome 18
performance test 84
Pierre Robin syndrome 13
post-auricular myogenic response
    100–1
prematurity 16, 19, 46

pure tones 4, 31, 37

respiratory distress 19
retinitis pigmentosa 18
rhesus incompatibility 16, 19–20
RNID picture screening test 76
room acoustics 95–97

scarlet fever 16
septrin 14
smallpox 16
sound 1–4
    babies' responsiveness 34–7
    bandwidth 34–5
    distortion 27–8
    duration 1, 34
    frequency 1–2
        octave intervals 2
        range for speech 2, 28–34
    intensity 1
    interference 37
    loudness 1–4, 34
    measurements 91–7
    octave band analysis 96
    pitch 1–2
    pressure (sound pressure
        level) 1, 4
    reflections 37
    spectra 28–34
    standing waves 37
    stimuli 28–34
sound level meters 36, 91–7
speech tests of hearing 65–84
    co-operative test 65, 68
    Dodd's insert board 78
    four-toy eyepointing test 66
    Kendall toy test 78
    RNID picture screening test
        (Reed) 76
    Stycar hearing test 75
    toy discrimination test
        (McCormick) 78–84
stapedial reflex 102
stroke 17
Stycar hearing test 75
syndromes 13–18
    Alport's 18
    Apert's 13
    branchio oto-renal 18

Cockayne 18
Crouzon's 13, 18
Down's 18
Goldenhar's 13
Hunter's 18
Klippel-Feil 13, 18
Pendred's 18
Pierre Robin 13
Treacher-Collin's 13, 17
Usher's 18
Waardenburg 17

toy discrimination test
(McCormick) 78–84
Treacher-Collin's syndrome 13,
17

tympanic membrane 9–10,
13–14
incision 14
mobility 102
perforated 13
retraction pocket 16

Usher's syndrome 18

van der Hoeve's disease 13

Waardenburg syndrome 17
warble tones 35–7
warbler 35–6, 56–7, 85–6
positioning 57